Praise for *The Diet Fix*

"I doubt you need anyone to tell you that 'dieting' is badly broken; just look around! But if you would like to know how to fix it and adopt a sensible, sustainable, and satisfying approach to weight control, then you certainly do need to hear from Dr. Yoni Freedhoff. In *The Diet Fix*, Dr. Freedhoff draws upon his excellent knowledge of relevant research and his many years of clinical experience to serve up empowering insights that are as much about living well as they are about losing weight. This is a terrific book."

> —David L. Katz, founding director of Yale University's Prevention
> Research Center and author of *Disease-Proof: The Remarkable Truth
> About What Makes Us Well*

"*The Diet Fix* is the real deal: a book that challenges the conventional wisdom about losing weight. This compassionate and hope-filled guide serves up the secrets to achieving—and maintaining—the weight that's right for you. Forget the quick fix: *The Diet Fix* will give you the tools you need to (finally) make peace with food."

> —Ann Douglas, author of *The Mother of All Pregnancy Books*

"Few people know as much about weight loss as Dr. Yoni Freedhoff. It is no surprise that he has produced a book that is the perfect combination of evidence-based facts and good, solid, usable advice. There is so much misinformation in the media about dieting. And so many trendy and near-useless diets. *The Diet Fix* is exactly what we need: a science-informed—and fun to read—road map to long-term weight loss success."

> —Tim Caulfield, author of *The Cure for Everything: Untangling Twisted
> Messages About Health, Fitness, and Happiness*

"After reading Dr. Freedhoff's book, I can conclude that only an expert who has real-life experience treating patients suffering with weight issues could have written this guide to weight management. Dr. Freedhoff distills the science of dieting into a very easy and practical read with proven results. Anybody who is battling weight issues should turn off their computer, get off the blog sites boasting miraculous weight loss, and just read this book."

> —Garth Davis, MD, medical director of bariatric surgery at Memorial Herman Hospital and author of *The Expert's Guide to Weight-Loss Surgery*

"*The Diet Fix* is a no-nonsense approach to realistic weight management by a recognized expert in the field. This step-by-step guide to long-term weight management provides the evidence, debunks common myths, and is chock-full of practical tips—the ultimate diet book for anyone wanting to stop dieting and start living."

> —Arya M. Sharma, MD/PhD, Disc. (h.c.), FRCPC, professor of medicine at the University of Alberta, Canada

"Dr. Yoni Freedhoff passionately demonstrates in *The Diet Fix* that he is every dieter's advocate. His 10-Day Reset will not only make you healthier, but it will also turn you into an activist around your own health."

> —James Beckerman, MD, author of *The Flex Diet*

THE
Diet Fix

WHY DIETS FAIL AND HOW TO MAKE YOURS WORK

Yoni Freedhoff, MD, CCFP, Dip. ABOM

HARMONY BOOKS
NEW YORK

Copyright © 2014 by Dr. Jonathan Freedhoff

All rights reserved.
Published in the United States by Harmony Books, an imprint of the Crown Publishing Group, a division of Random House LLC, a Penguin Random House Company, New York.
www.crownpublishing.com

Harmony Books is a registered trademark and the Circle colophon is a trademark of Random House LLC.

Library of Congress Cataloging-in-Publication data is available upon request.

ISBN 978-0-8041-3757-7
eBook ISBN 978-0-8041-3758-4

Printed in the United States of America

Jacket design by Jess Morphew

10 9 8 7 6 5 4 3 2 1

First Edition

For the four wonderful women in my life—
Stacey, Talia, Leah, and Yael

Contents

Contents

The Recovery

Preface

Whether it was Rita Mae Brown or Albert Einstein who first said it, the quote "Insanity is doing the same thing over and over again and expecting different results" might just as well have been written to describe society's past few hundred years of weight loss efforts. From the famous "milk cure" of the early 1800s, when dieters traveled deep into the Swiss Alps for the privilege of being assigned their own personal cow whose freshly milked udders provided their sole source of sustenance for 7 to 14 days, to William Banting's blockbuster 1864 bestseller *Letter on Corpulence*, to the 1970s 700-calorie Scarsdale Diet, grapefruit diets, and cabbage soup diets, there's certainly not been any shortage of traumatic diets over the years. The modern day isn't much different; for every ridiculous diet that falls out of favor, a new ridiculous diet is born. While all of these diets have markedly different methods of calorie control, they all share a common theme: in order to lose weight, you have to suffer. There is an underlying belief that success resides in white-knuckle willpower, in undereating, overexercising, and somehow learning to like it. These ideas are echoed not just by individuals, but by the media, the entertainment industry, and even our public health officials and allied health professionals.

So do any dieters succeed in not just losing, but in actually keeping it off?

A recent poll revealed that of the two-thirds of us who have medically significant amounts of weight to lose, nearly 60 percent have tried more than six times to lose weight.[1] Of those who've tried more than six times, 34 percent report having tried more than *20 times*, and 66 percent of those report *they've tried so many times they've lost count!*

What is it about how we're dieting that leads us, seemingly regardless of our chosen dietary approaches, to keep failing? Sure, you can point to various diets that have helped you lose weight, but why hasn't any diet been shown to help people uniformly keep it off? You might think that after literally centuries of different diets, at least one or two of them would have hit that mark. How is it possible that so many divergent approaches to dieting could fail so many people? From low-fat to low-carb, and from macrobiotic vegan to paleo, you'd think that given the incredible variety of approaches, if there were such a thing as the "right" diet, or the "best" diet, one of them would have led not only to significant losses, but also to their lifelong maintenance.

Truly, success with dieting must be measured by a diet's ability to help dieters keep their weight off, and not by simply the losing. But what if it's not the foods involved in the diets themselves that is tripping dieters up? Could there be some underlying collective feature that, despite their incredibly different recommendations, ties low-fat to low-carb; Ornish to Atkins? Some shared narrative that leads even those who successfully lose a great deal of weight on any given diet plan to abandon their efforts and eventually find themselves right back where they started—or worse yet, having gained back more than they'd lost in the first place?

Those were the questions nagging at me back in 2001 when I began my medical career as a physician with a traditional family practice in Canada's capital. Somewhere in the neighborhood of 65 to 70 percent of my patients struggled with excess weight, and a great many of them wanted to lose. With North America's $60 billion commercial weight loss industry, they had no shortage of diets or weight loss programs to consider, and they'd often ask me which diet or program they should try. Unfortunately, I had no wise answers. The thing is, medical schools and residencies don't adequately train doctors to provide thorough, helpful, and actionable advice regarding weight management or nutrition.[2] That's a strange thing, too, as diet and weight-related diseases have taken over from smoking as our number one preventable causes of death, and we doctors, well, death's the primary thing we're supposed to be trying to at least delay.

Given the myriad of medical conditions relatable to weight; the impact of weight on chronic disease, longevity, and quality of life; and the vast number of people asking me what to do, I realized that I had an obligation to my patients to try to understand weight management well enough to provide them with some useful, actionable advice. So despite having already spent more of my life in school than out, and thinking that my days of hard-core learning and studying were over, I embarked upon another chapter of education: obesity medicine.

I was absolutely amazed at what I found, and it was immediately apparent that weight was an incredibly complicated characteristic. From a survival standpoint, weight is life. Up until very recently, evolutionarily speaking, we've had to survive in the face of extreme dietary insecurities. You couldn't just buy sandwiches at your local gas station, and there was no phone number to call to have a pizza delivered. So when there were times of plenty, our bodies stored calories as fat for the floods, winters, and droughts that plagued our less-food-secure past, when eating was anything but a certainty. Consequently, aside from breathing, eating is our most important survival skill, and perhaps not surprisingly, after hundreds of millions of years of evolution, our bodies are finely tuned to ensure that we do survive. From hormones to gut peptides, our physiology actively protects us against ice ages and famines that in the grand scheme of time and genes occurred only moments ago, by generating hunger, and priming our brains' reward centers to seek out food much in the same way drug addicts' brains prime them to seek out their drug of choice. So it should not be a surprise that, in a sense, when faced with a situation where weight is lost, like for instance when someone goes on a diet, evolution fights back whereby our bodies are patently designed to try to preserve our remaining energy stores—our fat—making weight loss more difficult and weight gain that much easier.

What struck me, too, was the incredible variety of approaches to weight loss reported upon in the medical literature. While every approach had its own success stories, every approach also had its fair share of scientific opponents. From a practical and functional perspective, there truly didn't seem to be any "best" diet or "best" approach; every approach saw at least some success. But sadly, regardless of how their weight was lost, for the majority its regain was almost inevitable.

But there was one group who didn't regain: the group in the National

Weight Control Registry. Now, this wasn't a particular diet program. There were no "Registry Weight Loss Centers" in suburban strip malls, and no bestselling book backing them up. The registry was something akin to a club, where the sole requirement for membership was having maintained the loss of a significant amount of weight, regardless of how that weight was lost in the first place. Established in 1994 by Brown University School of Medicine's Rena Wing and University of Colorado's Jim Hill, the registry tracks individuals who've maintained a 30-or-more-pound weight loss for one or more years. Currently, there are over 10,000 registrants, the average of who has lost 67 pounds and kept them off for five and a half years! Clearly, these people are amazingly good at what they do, and they also serve as living, breathing testaments to the fact that keeping the weight off *is* doable. What's truly fascinating is that while the registrants used dozens of different approaches to lose their weight, they share a great many similarities in keeping it off.[3] These weight loss masters are more likely to plan their meals, track their intake, exercise, weigh themselves, and have breakfast. It seemed like a no-brainer; if I could simply teach my patients the skills the weight loss masters agree are required to keep the weight off, then they would enjoy the masters' same success. Only they didn't, but I'm getting ahead of the story.

In late 2003, my brother-in-law's close friend began what I thought to be a medically unsound program and my brother-in-law asked me, "Can you design a better one?" It was in that instant that I realized my life was about to change. Unhesitatingly, I said "Yes," and it was then that I set out to design and found the Bariatric Medical Institute.

In our institute's early days, I did what the evidence base said I should. I set a "medically significant" weight loss target of 10 percent for everyone who walked in the door; recommended that patients replace one, if not two, daily meals with a high-protein, medical-grade meal replacement; had patients keep food diaries; provided counseling with registered dietitians; encouraged and included exercise; promoted breakfast; scheduled regular weigh-ins; provided frequent follow-ups—and away we went.

On paper, the patients did fine. They lost weight and in many cases they even improved their health to the point of coming off some medications. They generally felt quite positive about the changes they were making in their lives. But they weren't uniformly satisfied. Although they lost enough weight to improve their qualities of life, their behavior changes were often short-lived, and many regained their lost weight and reverted to their old lifestyles over the course of the next one to two years.

Flash forward nine years, 13,500 hours, and nearly 40,000 one-on-one patient interactions, and our program and, more important, my philosophy have changed rather drastically. In the coming chapters, I'll lay out everything I've learned about long-term weight management, but in a nutshell, the main thing that was missing in those early days?

It was prescriptions for chocolate.

The Reveal

A (VERY) BRIEF HISTORY OF DIETING

Diets are anything but new. The first popular diet was a low-carb diet written by a British coffin maker in 1863. His name was William Banting, and the diet he championed and detailed in his *Letter on Corpulence, Addressed to the Public* was of the low-carb variety with an emphasis on eating meat, greens, and fruit while avoiding sugar, starches, dairy, and beer. His book was so incredibly popular that at the time, the word *banting* was used in conversation in place of *dieting*. Believe it or not, the book is still in print and you can even buy it in Kindle format. But it's been over the past 50 or so years, not coincidentally the time period in which obesity rates have nearly quadrupled, that the number of diets has grown by multiple orders of magnitude. At the time I'm writing this paragraph, over on Amazon there are over 37,000 books in their "diets and weight loss" racks.

Their strategies may all vary wildly, but ultimately we can subdivide all diet books and programs into seven broad categories:

1. Good/bad diets: These are among the simplest to follow. They have very clear rules that either cut out entire categories of foods or provide very specific meal plans. People on these types of diets are told that they don't need to track intake in terms of calories; instead they're told to avoid virtually an entire food group and they'll do fine. The most obvious examples of these are the ultralow-fat diet of Dr. Dean Ornish and the ultralow-carb diet of Dr. Robert Atkins.

2. Scientific and pseudoscientific diets: Rather than vilify an entire food group, these diets tend to focus only on specific foods within the group. Beans are good, carrots are bad. Oatmeal is good, rice is bad, and so on. Some, like the GI diet and the various surging paleo diets, are built on true scientific principles; others, like the blood type diet, and Suzanne Somers' food combination diet, tend to lapse into what might be described as common sense or intuitive, but are not in fact rooted in a rigorous, scientifically defensible evidence base.

3. Counting diets and programs: Food gets assigned points (or calories) and you're allotted a certain number with the aim of not going over. Perhaps the first counting diet was that of Dr. Lulu Hunt Peters, whose 1918 book, *Diet and Health, with the Key to the Calories,* was the first to recommend tracking calories. At the time, no one had heard of calories, and early on in the book Dr. Peters had to explain to readers how to pronounce the word. Of course, as far as counting diets go, there's no doubt that the grand champion is Weight Watchers, which in 50 years has enrolled tens of millions of people in more than 30 countries.

4. Crash diets: From the get-go, this type of diet is meant to be temporary. These diets aren't meant to be a "for good" solution but rather just a "for now" solution. Often they're undertaken as a way to lose weight before a particular event—a wedding, a trip, a high school reunion. They're usually massively restrictive, and the aim is to lose the weight to get to the event and then start eating again. Generally, they just involve eating very little of anything and sometimes as much as you want of just one very specific thing. The cabbage soup diet, the grapefruit diet, and the so-called master cleanse (that modified juice fast based on lemon juice and cayenne pepper) are this category's most obvious examples.

5. Exercise diets: These aren't necessarily diets so much as they are aggressive exercise programs undertaken with the expectation of weight loss. Invariably, the exercise is either highly intense (like boot camps, for instance) or exceedingly lengthy, sometimes even involving hours of daily activity.

6. Magic diets: Simply pop a magic pill or potion, or sidle up to some new-fangled exercise contraption, and presto chango, with zero effort and zero dietary change, the weight will just melt off. While I'm guessing magic diets aren't going to help melt weight, I'm positive they'll help melt bank accounts.

And then, of course, there's the most common and the most popular diet in history. The one diet that virtually anyone who has ever been unhappy or concerned about their weight has tried on at least one occasion. There's no book to read, or guru to follow. I call it the "Eat Smarter diet."

7. Eat Smarter diet: Honestly, who hasn't tried this one at least once? Even folks who aren't concerned about their weight have likely tried to "watch what they eat," "eat smarter," "be more aware," "be more thoughtful"—with the dual aims of "eating less" and "being more healthy." No books to purchase. No programs to consult. Just "eat less and exercise more" and "be smarter." And while it certainly makes sense and reflects the truism of energy balance, our bodies and our environment conspire to make this approach almost invariably useless.

"DOC, WHICH DIET SHOULD I GO ON?"

Is there one right diet for you? Is there some test you could take where you'd plug in your lifestyle, personality, and dietary preferences and out would come your perfect answer? If only it were that simple.

There are just so many variables. Some may be modifiable, but others simply aren't. It would be no easier to give yourself a palate that loves spinach and hates chocolate than it would be to swap out your genes. And don't kid yourself into thinking those things don't matter—they do. As the father of three beautiful little girls, I can tell you I sure had a great deal more free time to cook, sleep, and exercise before they came into my life. And although I know I'd probably be healthier if my favorite guilty pleasures were organic vegetables, I just can't seem to convince my mouth not to adore pizza, wings, burgers, and potato chips.

At the end of the day, all diets work, every last one. Even diets with nonsensical approaches can help people lose weight. But losing, of course, isn't the issue. I hear it all the time in my office and it's absolutely true: "Losing weight is easy; it's keeping it off that's hard."

So is there a common theme that makes keeping lost weight off difficult? Absolutely, and putting it simply, the common theme that makes long-term success difficult is the notion that suffering is a prerequisite to success.

TRAUMATIC DIETING

The questions people ask themselves when failing any given diet may sound familiar to you: *Why can't I just stick with it? What's wrong with me? What's my problem? Why am I such a failure?* It's the "it's not you, it's me" speech we give when we break up with someone, only unlike our breakups, where the statement's usually a sugarcoated lie, with weight management, we believe it. We failed, not our approach. *It's not the diet, it's me.*

If that's really true—that it's not the diet but rather us—how is it that failure is the norm? Can it really be that the past 50 years have seen a global pandemic loss of willpower? That somehow as a species we've become powerless to resist weight gain? That as individuals we simply can't control ourselves?

Maybe it's not you.

I'd be willing to wager that if you've been battling your weight for a while, you've invested more willpower in weight loss than in virtually any other area of your life. You've probably undertaken various white-knuckle diets, have set your alarm clock for 5:00 a.m. so that you can hit the treadmill downstairs, and you've likely eaten more salads and grilled boneless, skinless chicken breasts than you'd care to admit. You might have been on your first diet before you even made it to high school, and you may well have a veritable library of contradictory diet books filling shelves of your bookcase. Clearly, you've got willpower. So what is your problem? Why can't you "just stick with it"?

Human nature. We're just not built to needlessly suffer forever. Yes, we're an exceedingly adaptable species, but if the need to suffer isn't there, and if the alternative to suffering is easily accessible, like water seeking its own level, that's where your human nature and actual physiology will take you.

While there are those who will argue the scientific merits of one dietary approach over another until they're blue in the face, at the end of the day if you don't like the life you're living while you're losing weight, you're virtually certain to gain it back. Putting dietary theory aside, what we choose to put on our plates reflects a sort of personal homeostasis— meaning that while we put as much food on our plates as we feel we need to be satisfied, satisfaction isn't simply meeting some sort of stomach-filling need. Yes, there are our physiologically driven needs to satisfy our bodies' fuel requirements, but there are many other needs at work: our psychologically driven need to satisfy pleasure-related desires; our medical need for food to help us cope with stress or depression through its impact on cortisol; our hedonic need, in which food plays a genuinely celebratory role such as on vacations, birthdays, and holidays. So while one particular dietary regime may do a fabulous job on one area of need, if another need is left lacking, human nature being what it is, we're not likely to stay on program. It just isn't meeting our needs.

If you were to take a straw poll of your friends, family, and self, I'd bet that their answer to the question of what's required for long-term success is some variation on suffering, stick-to-it-iveness, or willpower; that success is therefore the by-product of willfully denying ourselves enjoyment and satisfaction from food. I disagree. To succeed in the long term, to actually keep the weight you lose off, I think you need to genuinely like your life with fewer calories.

Indeed, since time immemorial, dieting has been steeped and forged in suffering. Diets have been designed to be traumatic. They're about denial and sacrifice. They're about suffering and restriction. They're "die" with a "t."

And people wonder why they fail?

I think people fail because most diets promote an almost religious experience, whereby adherents are taught to all but shout, "Hear O world!

There are no other diets before mine." Dieters are expected to stick to a strict set of commandments, from "Thou shall not consume carbs" to "Thou shall honor thy treadmill and free weights." Transgressions against the diet are framed as being almost sinful, leaving dieters with a real sense of guilt over a plate of pasta. I hear about this guilt and regret all the time from my patients, so much so that I've come to think of the rules they are trying to follow as the deadly sins of dieting. I count seven most common misbeliefs, seven deadly dieting sins that have been championed by society as the necessary evils of success, and that while challenging and unpleasant, by society's misguided definition of *success*, need to be willfully endured forevermore. They're continually nurtured as necessities by popular culture, diet books, the entertainment and media industries, and even by allied health professionals. And while society believes them to be essential to success, I believe them to be integral to failure. In the next chapter, I'll tell you what they are.

DIETING'S SEVEN DEADLY SINS

Have you ever succumbed to the allure of dietary zealotry and felt so constrained by the rules of your regime that transgressions felt akin to sinning? While there may well be tens of thousands of different diets out there, dieting's seven deadly sins span their gamut, and though they may not all be present in each and every diet, I'm guessing that if you've battled with diets over the years, you're all too familiar with this motley collection, whereby your job was to endure and cultivate one or more of these and where failing to do so was a dietary sin.

1. HUNGER

"If I'm not hungry, my diet's not working."

Now, in my mind, the word *hungry* means a couple of different things. I use the word to describe not only the physical pit-of-your-stomach sensation of hunger (stomach hunger), but also simple cravings (head hunger). Purists and researchers might well disagree with my combination of what they in turn would refer to as *appetite* and *hunger,* but given that my experience has been that both head and stomach hunger respond identically to treatment, I think they're simply flip sides of the same coin. I've also met hundreds and hundreds of individuals who tell me that while they never experience stomach hunger, head hunger's a common and unwelcome visitor that manifests itself either as incredible cravings or as compulsive can't-stop-once-started eating.

Eating and drinking are second only to breathing in the hierarchy of survival needs, and after 100 million years of evolution, hunger is an extremely powerful physiologic drive. If you don't eat, you die. Taking one step back in time, if your cave-dwelling ancestors weren't great about eating as voluminously as possible when they were hungry and food was available, they might have had difficulty living long enough to pass on their genetic materials. Hunger is evolutionarily protective, and satisfying hunger when food is available has allowed our species to thrive.

However, over the course of the past hundred or so years, we've seen incredible changes to our food supply. There's no longer any dietary whim that can't be satisfied in a matter of moments, and where we once had to physically hunt for our food, now we simply have to dial for it. I think what we're seeing today in terms of societal weight struggle is reflective of the fact that our genes and physiology, honed over thousands of years of extreme dietary insecurity, still function as if the next meal might never come. While a thorough discussion of how our ancient physiology responds to hunger isn't necessary, it's worth a brief visit given its role in getting in the way of our best intentions.

From neuropeptides, to hormones produced by our actual fat cells, to proteins produced by our intestines, there are pathways and backup pathways whose jobs are to ensure that we eat enough to survive. There's leptin, produced by our own fat cells; its job is to act on the hunger center of our brains, the hypothalamus, where it inhibits appetite by signaling the brain that the body has had enough to eat. There's ghrelin, produced by our stomachs; it works in our hypothalamus too, but its job is to tell us to eat. There's neuropeptide Y, produced by the hypothalamus itself; its job is to decrease the expression of a gene that encodes for the production of proopiomelanocortin, a polypeptide that plays a role in appetite. It also decreases the synthesis of the pituitary hormone that signals the thyroid to make its hormone. There's peptide YY, produced by our small intestines, which decreases gut movement and the production of ghrelin, and acts in our brain's hunger center. And these are just the tip of our body's hunger system iceberg. It's a very complicated place and the problem is, those peptides, hormones, and proteins? They're still cave dwellers, and what once was a protective behavior—eating highly caloric foods in large quantities in response to hunger—has become in our modern day a kid-in-a-candy-store environment, and, at least in terms of weight, a liability.

And so dieters are taught that they must not be allowed to satisfy their cravings. But is that realistic? In the short run, maybe. After all, who hasn't white-knuckled through hunger during a diet's early days. But to have to white-knuckle cravings for life . . . well, that's a setup for failure. Consider this: recent functional brain scans have demonstrated that the very same areas of the brain that light up when we're craving foods are the ones that light up in drug addicts when they're craving their fix.[1] The difference between food and drugs? If you quit drugs, the brain pathway that's screaming for a hit will slowly quiet down. But you're not about to quit eating. Those pathways are here to stay and if you're hungry, they sure aren't going to be quiet.

So what do traumatic dieters do when they're hungry? Sometimes they may try to substitute "healthy" foods in the desired food's place, go for a walk, knit, call a friend, or otherwise try to distract themselves. But even if you successfully distract yourself for a few hours, cravings have a bad habit of coming back.

Ultimately, if your diet includes regular battles with hunger—whether it's head hunger and cravings or stomach hunger—my experiences with thousands of patients has taught me it is just a matter of time before you end up giving in. There are 100 million years of evolution telling you what to do, and while you might be able to beat your urges from time to time, eventually (you and I both know) they're going to win.

2. SACRIFICE

"No, no birthday cake for me, thanks."

There is a widespread belief that success in dieting depends on your ability to make sacrifices. Perhaps you'll feel the need to turn down invitations to social events, or to forgo cake at a birthday party, or to always be the designated driver so as to avoid those pesky alcohol calories. Yet celebrating with food is part of the human condition—literally, from births to deaths and everything in between, food is used by our species to mark important occasions. From formal and traditional holiday meals like Christmas turkey with all the fixings to pulling out all the stops when we entertain our friends and colleagues, to having our indulgent favorites on our birthdays, food often plays a starring role in our lives' various events.

Perhaps it's this weaving of food into the social fabric of humanity that inevitably leads folks who are blindly restricting various foods to "give in to temptation." Whether it's a vacation, a wedding, a religious holiday, a birthday, or just such a long time since they let themselves have a night out with friends, traumatic dieters will inevitably relax their restrictions, often in a "write-off" manner. Understandably, given the pleasure they receive from their social meals and relaxed rules, when life grinds back to a more boring normal, it's difficult for them to get back to their blindly restrictive, sacrificial lifestyles—and oftentimes, they don't. It's also important to remember that those shared meals play a role in maintaining our real-life social networks, and while I'm a huge fan of virtual social networks, I'm pretty sure that food is undoubtedly the oldest and most profound social networking tool we've got.

While discretionary compromises are clearly required in our Willy Wonkian food environment, regularly and blindly sacrificing the social pleasures of food in the name of weight management virtually guarantees the abandonment of whatever weight management strategy you're employing. Sometimes you just need to be able to kick back with your friends and relatives. Putting it a bit more plainly: if your life includes an easily avoidable area of perpetual sacrifice, there's little to no likelihood you'll be willing to live with that perpetual sacrifice forever—and that's not a statement about you as a person, it's just a reflection of our shared human nature.

3. WILLPOWER

"If I close my eyes and run past the cupboard,
I can make it to the bedroom without hitting the chips."

We eat according to our three basic dietary needs: physiologic needs, which are about satisfying that primal drive for fullness and fuel; psychological needs, which consciously or unconsciously involve our use of food as a medication to decrease our bodies' stress hormones and in so doing at least temporarily improve and calm our mood; and hedonic needs, which is where we eat purely because we can and purely because food tastes good. Meaning that whatever we're eating before we start our diets, we're eating the exact amount that meets those three distinct though perhaps occasionally overlapping needs. While dieting theory suggests that we should simply be able to will ourselves to need less, to resist our temptations, if our needs are no longer being met, even if it's "just" our hedonic needs, eventually we'll give in.

But why? Why can't we resist temptations forever if that is what it takes to reach health or weight loss goals? Perhaps one of the reasons we can't resist forever is that we have only a limited amount of resistance or willpower to draw upon each day; when we've used it up, it's gone. That was the theory of a researcher from Florida State University named Roy Baumeister. In the late 1990s, he and his colleagues set up a series of experiments that demonstrated just how real this phenomenon was, including one in which subjects were asked to resist eating chocolate and cookies and in their place choose radishes.[2] What Baumeister and his team found was that in a subsequent task that involved trying to solve what was actually an impossible puzzle, the folks who had resisted the allure of the cookies gave up sooner. In a very real sense, they ran out of resistance or self-control sooner.

And it might be that we're not only limited in our total amount of daily willpower, but also in our minute-to-minute use of what we've got. In 1999, researchers Baba Shiv out of the University of Iowa and Alexander Fedorikhin out of Washington State University devised a simple experiment.[3] Students were given either two- or seven-digit numbers to memorize and then were asked to walk down the hall where they were offered two different snack choices: chocolate cake or fruit salad. Amazingly, the students who were trying to remember seven digits who identified themselves as impulsive were found to be twice as likely to choose the chocolate cake as the folks trying to remember two digits, leading the authors to conclude that a larger "cognitive load" made resisting the less healthy snack more challenging. Given how much each of us has going on in our daily lives, it's a small wonder we aren't constantly eating chocolate cake.

What Baumeister, Shiv, and Fedorikhin have demonstrated is that resistance is both finite and partly indivisible. Truth be told, we have a limited pool of willpower to draw upon; once it's gone, it's gone, and we don't share it particularly well between tasks, which perhaps is why at the end of the day, resistance is indeed futile.

4. BLIND RESTRICTION

"The only way to lose weight is to kick this
(insert food or food group here) out of my life!"

There is a simple rule that many traumatic dieters believe: *I'm not allowed to eat* _____, where the blank applies to either specific "danger" foods or entire food groups or categories. For most this leads to a perception of some foods as their "danger" foods—foods of which they believe a single bite will lead to out-of-control bingeing.

Could there be some truth to this one? Aren't some food groups healthier than others, and can anyone really be trusted with an open bag of Oreos?

There will always be those who preach that certain food groups are less healthy than others; low-carb advocates will suggest you markedly restrict carbohydrates, paleo advocates will suggest you avoid dairy and grains, and true fad diets might have you avoid combining certain foods or food groups together.

Some of these recommendations may well have real scientific reasoning to back them up, while others will just have pseudoscientific bafflegab that more often than not sounds logical but lacks actual clinical supporting evidence.

But is eating really only about health or weight management? Do our palates use scientific literature as their litmus tests for their desires? Of course not. Food's not just fuel. If it were, we'd all swallow our calorie pills, followed by our vitamin pills, and be whatever weight we wanted as we could simply take in more or less calories as we saw fit.

Food is a great many things, and while I know that "danger" foods can truly be dangerous to people's best intentions, I'm quite certain that a plan that has the dieter thinking *I can't eat chocolate* will eventually lead them right back to the lifestyle they had before they decided they couldn't be trusted around one of life's most delicious pleasures.

Food can't simply be about fuel or sustenance; food must be allowed to comfort, celebrate, bolster, and support. Like it or not, life includes chocolate, and later in this book, I'll be teaching you how to include it along with all of your other "danger" foods.

5. SWEAT

"You have to sweat, and sweat a lot. Bonus points if you feel like puking."

Plenty of people are taught that the magic bullet of weight loss is to simply "eat less and move more." Worse, many people believe that exercise, an incredibly enjoyable and healthful behavior, must be taken to unenjoyable extremes if weight is a concern.

Popularized by television shows like *The Biggest Loser*, and exploited by the food industry to shift the focus off of their products, the belief that our struggles with weight are due to inactivity is perhaps so readily accepted because it seems so intuitive. My friend and colleague Dr. Arya Sharma, the scientific director of the Canadian Obesity Network, has dubbed this belief "ELMM Street" (eat less, move more), and in my opinion this notion can definitely become a nightmare!

Of course, intuition isn't always accurate, and the results of studies designed to look at whether as a whole society has slowed down over the course of these past 30 years and consequently gained weight might surprise you. The gold standard method of measuring our activity levels involves using radioactively labeled water to determine exactly how much energy we're expending. Using this technique, researchers have determined that despite obesity rates doubling since 1980, our energy expenditures have remained the same.[4] We're just not moving less, and in fact some researchers believe that we're actually genetically programmed to move a specific amount, which might help to explain why studies comparing the energy expenditures of urban Chicago women to rural Nigerian women show no differences in total daily burn,[5] and why a study on one of the world's last hunter-gatherer societies—the Hadza—also was unable to find a demonstrable increase in energy expenditure.[6]

But so what? Even if we didn't get into this mess because we're moving less, can't we get out of it by moving more? Can't we as a society simply get more active and literally burn off the weight we've gained?

Probably not. The unfortunate truth is that exercise alone doesn't burn enough calories to be the whole solution for society's weight woes.

To lose one pound a week through exercise would require most people to endure seven hours of weekly brow-bursting exercise, seven hours of sweaty treadmills, ellipticals, body pump classes, and Zumba. And what if during that week you decided that "because you exercised" you were entitled to a larger portion of cake, an extra beer, or an indulgent meal out as a reward? What if "because you exercised" you were hungry and needed a larger portion to feel full? Or if you took the advice of that poster on the gym wall that told you to drink chocolate milk to help with your so-called recovery or refueling? Well, if you do any of those things, you can kiss the caloric benefits of your exercise and sweat good-bye. As for that "recovery" beverage, it probably contains 30 sweaty minutes' worth of exercise calories. Exercise alone isn't sufficient. You just can't outrun your fork.

That doesn't mean exercise doesn't play a role in weight management. It's just that exercise alone, or exercise undertaken to compensate for an indulgent diet, is almost certain to fail. Overexercising is as much a risk to dieters as undereating. For those who equate success with extremes of sweat, stopping excessive exercise understandably often leads them to the abandonment of their dietary efforts as well. I'd bet it's a rare dieter who hasn't abandoned at least one of their weight loss efforts when their movement in the gym didn't seem to translate into movement on the scale.

But even with those exercisers who do see their scales move, exercising past the point of enjoyment will lead anyone to eventually stop exercising. A grueling workout performed most days of the week might allow you to lose weight, but at a certain point life will get in the way. Whether because of exhaustion, injury, scheduling problems, boredom, or other reasons, every diet that includes extreme exercise runs the risk of getting benched when excessive exercise naturally and understandably falls by the wayside.

6. PERFECTIONISM

"I have to be perfectly perfect or else I'll never lose weight."

Rationally, I'm fairly confident that everyone recognizes perfection to be a terrible goal. So why is it that so many people cling to the idea of dieting perfection as a personal identity?

Given the fact that real life includes chocolate, temptation, social pressures to eat, and a limited and finite pool of personal resistance, how well do you think a goal of dietary perfectionism will fare in the real world? Not so well, and yet I'm guessing many of you reading this book have fallen into the trap of perfectionism. A person who's down 35 pounds goes on a cruise, gains 5 pounds, and when they come back and step on a scale, they can't stop beating themselves up about those five when they could instead focus on being down 30. It's something I see regularly. Someone might set himself or herself a goal of losing a certain amount of weight per week or in total, and if they can't achieve every last pound of it, they ignore the success that they did achieve and instead give up wholly on trying. Or perhaps they've set out to keep a food diary but realize they've missed part of their day and then put it off until tomorrow, or even the next Monday (after all, they have to have a complete week). Discounting everything you've accomplished because of one imperfection leads perfectionists to "write-offs"—thinking that one solitary misstep means that the rest of the day is shot, so why not write it off further with highly indulgent bingeing?

Is there anything worthwhile in our life that doesn't come with setbacks? Our relationships, our jobs, our parenting, our health—none of them follow straight line patterns, and neither will weight management or healthy living efforts. Denying diets the ability to wax and wane is a recipe for perpetual waning.

At the end of the day, people who strive for perfection in long-term weight loss will disappoint themselves. And if faced with that disappointment too often, the likelihood is that they will end up giving up altogether.

7. DENIAL

"Nothing tastes as good as thin feels."

Every great love affair has a honeymoon period, and dieting's no exception. Perhaps as a consequence, the early days of any diet are the easiest. It doesn't matter how extreme the effort might be, how much restriction is involved, or how much hunger you might be facing; if the scale is moving, especially if it's moving quickly, it's easy to deny that you're suffering. I regularly see patients who are coming off the most extremes of dieting efforts—very low calorie diets, sometimes even involving injectable vitamins, hormones, and incredibly limited dietary options. Yet they'll often tell me that their restrictive diets were "great," and that they just failed to stick with them.

But if their diet really was so great, why couldn't they stick with it? Why wasn't "thin" enough to keep them restricting? In almost every case, the person on one of these intense diets gave it up once the scales slowed down. While their scales were regularly whispering sweet nothings in their ears, it was easy to live in denial of their actual suffering. After all, the numbers on that scale were flying down! But eventually and inevitably, their weight loss slowed down. And this is the problem with weight loss: it simply doesn't last forever. It slows down because as the body loses weight, physiologic changes called "metabolic adaptations" occur that are designed to protect us against what the body perceives as some sort of famine. It slows down because as we lose weight, there's literally less of us to burn calories. Weight loss also slows down because most people who go on diets, in the diet's early honeymoon-like days, are often much more vigilant and strict. Eventually, if the scale slows down too much, stops, or (worse) starts going back up, suddenly all of the suffering becomes too much for them to endure. After all, why suffer if there's no payoff?

DIETING'S SEVEN DEADLY TRAUMAS

Whether you're familiar with one or all of dieting's seven deadly sins, the consequent experience of guilt, frustration, sadness, and suffering associated with the sin's transgression can become traumatic. Perhaps it therefore follows that if there are seven deadly dieting sins, there are also seven deadly dieting traumas, deadly in the sense that they're going to kill your diet if you experience them for a prolonged period of time. These traumas are real, and it is an exceedingly rare dieter who hasn't experienced one or more of them consequent to their dieting efforts. It doesn't matter how smart a person may be, or how motivated they were when they started their diet; recurrently feeling traumatized will lead them to throw in the towel. While there are a great many different diets out there to choose from, it's these traumatic experiences that serve as the common thread that leads even their most dedicated dietary adherents to ultimately fail—and it's these common traumas that tie together even the most wildly divergent diets.

1. GUILT

CASE STUDY

Maryanne is a 39-year-old mother of two young girls. She's never thought of herself as skinny, though looking back on photos from her early years from school, she can't understand why she ever thought she'd been fat. "If I could only go back in time and tell the younger me how great I looked."

Maryanne has been through the gauntlet of weight loss efforts. Starting out with the simple and classic, "I'll just eat smarter and exercise more" diet, she progressed through Weight Watchers ("It worked the first time") to Nutrisystem, to self-help books, and finally to a doctor-supervised very low-calorie diet. "I actually didn't feel badly doing that one. I wasn't ever hungry. I just couldn't keep it up, and when I got to my goal and I started to try to enjoy food just a little, I couldn't believe how quickly the pounds came back on." She came to me because she'd had enough and wanted to learn how to live the life she wanted her daughters to live.

A short time into our program, Maryanne came into my office looking defeated. When I asked her how things were going, she answered "Terrible," and proceeded to tell me about how she'd indulged at her sister-in-law's wedding. "I blew it. I planned on just having a little bit of everything, and I was doing all right until dessert, but then when the dessert turned out to be a buffet, even though I told myself I was just going to take just two tiny chocolates, once I started, I couldn't stop."

After the wedding, Maryanne was despondent. She felt so guilty about what she'd eaten that she cried in her bathroom before going to bed. The next morning she decided she wasn't going to bother with breakfast because she'd eaten too many calories the night before. But by the time the evening rolled around, she'd gotten into the cereal, the peanut butter, and a few other foods she'd been denying herself in the hopes of finally losing weight for good. Feeling out of control, and with ever-growing guilt, the week that followed saw Maryanne abandoning all of her dietary and lifestyle strategies, and led her to all-too-familiar feelings of self-loathing and shame.

Maryanne's story isn't unique. The very idea of forbidden foods is a mainstay of people on traumatic diets, and they lead to very slippery guilt slopes. Have you ever felt so guilty about your dietary or healthy living choices that instead of trying to improve upon them, you simply gave up?

Given the unreasonable expectations of all of dieting's seven deadly sins, there's really no end to guilt. You may feel guilt over what you did or didn't eat, guilt over your lack of exercise, guilt over your weak will, guilt over that piece of birthday cake, guilt over going over your calories, guilt over exceeding your points, or guilt over not being able to simply will away your dietary desires. Guilt is the cornerstone of dieting's deadly traumas, it's unspeakably common, and it can wear us down until it has totally destroyed our motivation to stick with a plan. Certainly, it's not surprising that excessive or recurrent guilt decreases the likelihood of long-term success.

2. SHAME

CASE STUDY

Corrine is a 46-year-old married mother of two. She's struggled with her weight since she headed off to college, and she can't remember anymore how many diets she's tried over the years.

Corrine's husband is one of those folks who can eat whatever they want and never gain an ounce, and he doesn't understand her struggles. He regularly tells her that all she needs to do is go to the gym more and to eat less. Worse, he makes fun of her weight, not just when they're alone, but also in front of their children. Recently, her 100-pound 13-year-old daughter asked her if she thought she was fat.

Corrine tries to hide her eating from her husband. Sometimes she eats in the car on the way home; other times she waits until he's out to raid the cupboards. Corrine tells me that she and her husband are very rarely intimate and that she often gets dressed in the dark and actively avoids mirrors.

Corrine had lost 30 pounds with us when one day she arrived in my office in tears. She'd gone shopping for a new dress to wear to a party and had bought one that, unlike most of her wardrobe, didn't hide her curves. When she came down the stairs, her husband took one look at her and asked, "Are you really going to go out looking like that?"

Corrine was devastated. Here she had been proud of how she looked, and with one mean-spirited comment, she was completely deflated. She felt ashamed of herself for letting her husband's comment get to her, but at the same time she couldn't help but wonder if there weren't some truth to it; after all, she was still a size 14.

Corrine spiraled some after that. Overexercising, undereating, and then struggling with hunger and bingeing. It took more than six months for us to steer her back to trying to live a life she actually enjoyed, husband's snide comments be damned.

In a now classic study, Gary Foster and his colleagues looked at the weight loss desires of 60 women about to embark on a weight loss program, and those same women's actual outcomes.[1] The women were asked to detail how much weight they would need to lose in order to reach their own personally determined "goal" weight, as well as how much weight they felt they needed to lose to reach "dream," "happy," "acceptable," and "disappointed" degrees of weight loss. Remarkably, the average "goal" weight loss was 32 percent of their presenting body weight, and yet following the completion of the study, 47 percent of the women hadn't even lost enough weight to feel "disappointed." I would imagine instead many simply felt shame.

Have you ever felt so ashamed of your body or your weight that you took on a diet or lifestyle that you knew was completely over-the-top ridiculous? Have you ever quit a diet because you felt like you just did not have what it took to get results that would matter to yourself or to those around you? People set incredibly lofty weight loss goals for themselves, which isn't necessarily a bad thing. But if realistically the goals are unlikely ever to be reached, the tendency is for dieters to blame themselves and not their diets when they eventually quit. Rather than assume it was their choice of program, their body's physiology, or factors that come from their daily lives, people still assume that personal flaws are to blame for their lack of success.

The fact is, while there are certainly things you can change that will help you lose weight, there is no doubt there are other things affecting your weight that you either won't be willing or able to change, and here I'm not just talking about our incredibly obesogenic environment. Jobs, genetics, body frames, caregiving requirements, and dozens of other factors truly beyond your control do affect your weight. To put this more bluntly, life affects weight, and while we may all have weight loss dreams and goals, sometimes, even despite our very best efforts, real life prevents us from reaching them. Just as in every other area of life, there's a wide range of normal when it comes to weight. What's ideal for one person most assuredly won't be ideal for all. Not respecting the impact of your weight-related realities on your outcomes may lead you to feel personally ashamed at your inability to reach some preset numerical goal. In turn, that shame may lead you to quit altogether.

Unfortunately, people's traumatic dieting shame isn't relegated solely to their perceived lack of inner fortitude. It's also commonly reflected in shame surrounding their outward appearance. It may seem a bit paradoxical, but oftentimes when people lose weight, their body image decreases. Looking at yourself more frequently in the mirror to scrutinize the physical effects of a diet could actually lead you to feel less comfortable with your appearance than before you lost.

Poor body image often fuels self-doubt and self-loathing and unfairly robs people of the ability to take pride in their accomplishments. No doubt it's the deadly sin of perfectionism that fuels this dieting trauma.

3. FAILURE

CASE STUDY

Eunice is 66 years old and has struggled with weight her whole life. While she's had some intermittent successes and even served as a leader in her local Overeaters Anonymous chapter, she's still extremely frustrated with her weight. She retired three years ago with the hope of finally tackling her weight, and three years later, she found her way to my office.

Eunice's mother put her on her first diet at the age of eight, and she rode Eunice about her weight until the day she died. So did Eunice's first husband, whom she left over 25 years ago.

While Eunice is sometimes able to take a few steps forward in her weight loss efforts, she often finds herself sabotaging them.

As a traumatic dieter, it's Eunice's past dieting traumas that haunt her. Though it's not usually a conscious thought, she wonders whether the reason for her recurrent self-sabotage lies with her mother and ex-husband. In a sense, she doesn't want to succeed in losing, because if she did she'd be giving them a degree of satisfaction that their constant and painful derision simply doesn't deserve. Eunice truly struggles with her self-sabotage. She gets incredibly frustrated with herself. But to hear her tell it, if she doesn't bother trying, she doesn't need to be afraid of failing, because not trying and failing, while frustrating, isn't terrifying, whereas trying and failing—that means she's got no hope.

Have you failed so often at managing your weight that now you're afraid to truly try? Closely linked to guilt and shame is the trauma of failure. With the seven deadly dieting sins' hugely unrealistic goals and expectations come many inevitable failures that plague even those dieters who don't perpetually feel guilt, as they don't need to feel like they've done anything wrong to feel like a failure.

Frequently feeling like a failure may be more dangerous than simply feeling guilty. Failure can become part of a bigger picture and contribute to a belief that you're formatively and broadly flawed, not just with weight management, but with life in general. Oftentimes, this can lead to a self-fulfilling failure prophesy, whereupon even with thoughtful efforts, minor slips are rapidly and markedly magnified into complete collapses. This phenomenon might lead a person who has successfully lost a significant amount of weight, who over the course of real life gains back a few pounds, to feel as if they've accomplished nothing. They perceive themselves as "failing again," give up on themselves and their lifestyle changes, and then regain all of their lost weight.

4. DEPRESSION

CASE STUDY

Julie is 44 years old and recently divorced. Her husband spent much of their marriage berating her for her weight. While he walked his home like a beat cop on the lookout for food crimes, he himself ate junk food constantly and regularly suggested that they go out to eat.

For many years Julie reports struggling with extremely low self-esteem and poor body image. Since her divorce her mood has become even more of a challenge. She's been finding it difficult to concentrate at work, and has been having difficulty sleeping. Food is her comfort; she definitely considers herself to be an emotional eater.

Julie's family doctor recently put her on an antidepressant and a sleeping pill and since then, Julie has gained 20 pounds. She wonders whether it might be due at least in part to the medication.

Before coming to see me, Julie had been trying to diet but was failing miserably. She told me that she couldn't seem to "stay on track" for more than a day or two. She said that her inability to stay focused made her even more depressed. Though Julie was adamant that it was her weight that was making her depressed, I explained to Julie that intentional weight loss and life change had to take a backseat to treating her mood; to pursue lifestyle change in the midst of a major mood disturbance is neither wise nor fair. Julie's priority had to be getting her mood and her life back in order, and then and only then would it be fair for her to start trying to tackle her weight.

Following a few adjustments to her medications and some counselling, Julie's mood improved enough for her to start taking on organized lifestyle change. While it was not perfectly smooth sailing, with her renewed ability to concentrate and her improved insight, she and I were able to work through her rough patches.

Has your mood ever held you back from your best intentions? Depression itself makes organization, concentration, and planning much more difficult (and sometimes even impossible). And these are the very qualities most required to nurture and sustain intentional lifestyle change!

Ongoing mood disturbances may predispose a person to struggle with dietary control because food is physiologically comforting; eating food, especially indulgent, sugary foods, actually helps a person feel real relief.

Food has a truly medicinal role for folks struggling with mood, and if those folks then combine the emotional role of food as comfort with a traumatic and restrictive diet, the drive to eat will rise while the ability to stay in control will fall. While the impact of food on mood is complex, describing this maladaptive feedback loop is fairly straightforward: traumatic dieting leads to recurrent struggle, which in turn leads to worsening mood. Worsening mood affects our bodies' stress hormones and brain reward centers, and food helps to soothe those insults, worsening the struggle until eventually people give up the fight.

Depressed mood often leads to increased personal frustration, as sufferers don't recognize the fact that the mood disturbance itself makes organized behavior change challenging. In turn, struggles purely related to their mood disturbance are interpreted by the individual as further examples of their own personal failures with weight loss. These perceptions of failure then may fuel a shame spiral and an inevitable abandonment of that person's attempted lifestyle changes.

5. DESPAIR

CASE STUDY

George is a 38-year-old married, shift-working paramedic, and dad of a 12-year-old boy. George was an athlete in high school and even played college-level football, but once he stopped playing and started working, his weight rose rapidly. Lately, he's been feeling hopeless about the future and he's terrified that unless he does something soon, he'll never do anything.

George tells me he's embarrassed because as a health professional, he feels he ought to know better. He's also embarrassed because coaching his son's football team leaves him breathless just trying to keep up on the sidelines.

Exploring his motivation some, George admits that he's afraid. One of his colleagues recently had a heart attack at the age of 44, and heart disease is in George's family history. He wonders whether he might be diabetic, and tells me that he's been actively avoiding going to his family physician because he doesn't want to face that possibility.

I asked George whether he thought now was a good time to try to focus on lifestyle changes and he told me he wasn't sure. But he felt he needed to do something, and he can't seem to find the motivation because "I've just got so far to go."

Have you ever not taken that first step because the journey itself seemed too daunting? Could it have been because you couldn't stop thinking about how long the whole journey would take or how hard it would be? Despair is the very normal response to enduring recurrent negative emotions, including all of the aforementioned diet-induced traumas of guilt, shame, failure, and depression.

The fact is, food is both a comfort and a pleasure. Since humanity's earliest days, indulgent food has been a social lubricant and a vehicle to demonstrate and cultivate friendship, caring, and love. Food affects our hormones, decreasing stress in a real and formative manner. Is it any wonder then that losing the ability to maintain a normal, human, rewarding relationship with food is traumatic?

For traumatic dieters, food is often thought of as an enemy, and the pleasure and social lubrication it genuinely delivers become feared. These struggles lead to a sense of despair and the belief that their relationship with food will only ever be adversarial. Given food's roles in both comfort and celebration, when traumatically dieting for some that despair is akin to losing a close friend.

The other exceedingly common despair felt by traumatic dieters stems from feeling overwhelmed. Many people feel as though they have too much weight to lose before they can reach some idealized goal; they get stuck in the despair that they'll never achieve it or that it will take forever. I've even seen this happen following a truly successful loss, whereby a patient who had managed to easily and nontraumatically over the course of eight months lose 60 pounds and break out of the 300s suddenly felt overwhelmed by the fact that to reach her next goal of 199 pounds, even if all went great, might take her more than a year. She actually gained back

15 pounds at that point, before we were able to steer her back on course by helping her focus more on the journey than on the finish line.

6. BINGE EATING

CASE STUDY

Karen is a 32-year-old married bank teller. She's been trying to get pregnant for over two years and she was sent to our office by a local fertility doctor who wants her to lose 100 pounds before she can be considered a candidate for in vitro fertilization. Karen tells me that she's struggled with her weight her entire life, but after a few questions from me, admitted that really her weight struggles began at the age of eight after she was sexually assaulted by one of her uncles.

Though she doesn't think it was conscious at the time, she has no doubt now that her weight is her shield. It pushes away attention, and in a sense makes her invisible to the world.

Following her assault, she gained 40 pounds in just six months. At first her parents didn't say or do anything, but within a few years and after her continued gains, they started to practice tough love and dramatically restricted Karen's access to her favorite sugary treats.

As a teen, Karen would use her babysitting money and allowance to buy chocolate bars that she would secretly eat in her room late at night. Feeling ashamed, she suffered through a spell of bulimia for a few years. Once she hit college, the purging stopped but the bingeing continued.

Nowadays, Karen tells me, "I rarely eat breakfast and generally I try to have something healthy and small for lunch, knowing full well that on my drive home I'll be stopping by the 7-Eleven and a drive-thru, where I'll have at least three candy bars and two meal combos before getting home and joining my husband for dinner. If he's going to be out late, I'll often buy a pint of ice cream or a bag of cookies on the way home and plan to finish them long before he gets back." She also told me that every morning she sets out thinking today's going to be the day she doesn't follow through, that she's just going to drive straight home, and that every afternoon, pulling into the driveway, she hates herself a little bit more.

Karen's story is sadly not unique. The use of weight as a defense mechanism is not uncommon, and for some, losing weight triggers old anxieties as they start to receive more attention or compliments about how they look.

Binge eating disorder (BED) is by far the most common eating disorder around. Estimates have put 30 percent of folks seeking professional help with weight as suffering with binge eating disorder.[2]

Do you know what one of the most common triggers for binge eating is? Dietary restriction. I can't tell you how many folks I've seen who struggle with binge eating when their struggles began either during or immediately following an overly restrictive traumatic diet.

Of dieting's deadly traumas, binge eating is certainly one of the most psychologically devastating. People who binge describe themselves as feeling out of control; once an episode is over, they will often feel wracked with guilt, shame, and self-loathing. Worse, the tendency for many binge eaters is to believe that in order to beat their disorder, they simply need to become stricter with themselves. Danger foods are banned from homes, and activities are created to fill danger times—choices and flexibility diminish. Unfortunately, increasing the degree of restriction simply increases the desire to binge.

Should a person with a tendency towards binge eating believe success will ultimately require them to be severely strict, there's little doubt their efforts will be both painful and short-lived. They'll be painful while they white-knuckle through their urges, and they'll be short-lived as regularly white-knuckling by the cupboards—for anyone, let alone someone who struggles with binge eating—is next to impossible.

7. WEIGHT CYCLING AND METABOLIC SLOWDOWN

CASE STUDY

Steven is a high-powered 49-year-old executive with a local high-tech firm. He travels regularly, and as a consequence, eats out a great many meals. His pattern before coming to see me had been to recurrently enroll in an extremely aggressive and restrictive weight loss program. He'd come to see me now because after five rides on this yo-yo, he was now 80 pounds heavier than the first time he tried, as with each successive effort he regained more weight than he had lost.

When I measured his body fat percentage as part of our energy expenditure measurements, it was just north of 50 percent. Half of him was fat, more than double the body fat percentage of the average man his age.

I explained to Steven that his story and body fat percentage weren't surprising as each time he rapidly cycled his weight, his body likely experienced a dramatic loss of muscle mass, which along with the metabolic adaptations that occurred with each loss, in turn contributed to a cyclical slowing of his metabolism. Every time he would simply return to his pre–extreme weight loss lifestyle, not even eating one ounce more than before, superimposed on his ever slower metabolism he successively gained more and more weight.

Steven was quite uncomfortable with my recommendation that he might want to consider a slower approach to weight loss, and he told me he needed some time to think on things.

The more restrictively a person diets, the more likely they are to experience regular weight cycling. It's the yo-yo effect, but unlike a yo-yo, sometimes the upswing winds up at a higher location than where it started.

The biggest danger to aggressive weight cycling is metabolic slowdown. If a person undertakes an extremely restrictive diet, they're likely to lose a disproportionate amount of muscle—meaning that losing 50 pounds ultrarapidly will cause a greater loss of muscle and lean tissue than losing that same 50 pounds slowly. Muscle is responsible for a fair percentage of our total daily caloric burn, and is also of course responsible for much of our feelings of daily vigor and energy. Consequently, an ultrarapid 50-pound loss may lead a person to not only lose the actual strength to continue with their efforts, but also to suffer from a disproportionately slower metabolism consequent to their disproportionate loss of muscle and perhaps an amplified near-starvation adapted metabolic response. This phenomenon may help to explain why it is that people who lose large amounts of weight rapidly often regain more than they'd lost despite in fact not eating any more than they used to. If that person then goes back to the life they were living before their ultrarapid loss, even though they're not eating any more than they did prior to losing weight, they'll gain back more than they lost because their body now burns fewer calories than it used to. As well, the weight they gain back will primarily be fat, which is why body fat percentages often climb higher following a weight cycle. Weight cycling is commonplace among traumatic dieters, and with each cycle more and more lean tissue is lost, leading to slower and slower metabolisms and higher and higher weights.

And of course, gaining back more than you lost even once, well, that's a trauma unto itself.

What's truly astounding is the fact that the sins of dieting and their resulting traumas are not exactly unknown to dieters when they set out to diet—on the contrary. I'd wager that the majority of diet veterans know full well what lies in their next dieting trench. They'll tell you at their diet's outset that it's going to be difficult, that they're going to have to make sacrifices, that they're going to have to exercise a lot of willpower—maybe more than ever before. They'll tell you that if they "mess up" they're going to feel guilty, that they're worried about inevitable bingeing, and that they'll probably just throw in the towel after they've messed up or struggled enough. Truth be told, they know the futility of traumatic dieting. They've lived with traumatic diets time and time again. It's just that each and every time they muster up the courage for yet another diet, they've somehow managed to at least partially convince themselves *this time's going to be different.* But if the new diet book or guru's plan involves some combination of undereating, overexercising, blind restriction, and sacrifice, it's just going to end the same way.

POST-TRAUMATIC DIETING DISORDER

I f insanity is doing the same thing over and over again and expecting a different result, how can it be that we've all gone so mad? What makes intelligent, levelheaded people so irrational as to regularly and recurrently adopt dietary strategies and beliefs that in turn lead to diet-ending traumatic failures? Is it simple, recurrent, individualized desperation, or could it be that our collective insanity stems at least in part from forces beyond our individualized control? We're going to explore this, but before we do, let's take a few steps sideways to the field hospitals of World War I.

World War I launched a new era in warfare. Modern technology allowed for the massive mobilization of troops and provided the literal ammunition for incredible suffering, destruction, and death. Poison gas, artillery, tanks, and trenches—it was horrific, and by Armistice Day over nine million soldiers had been killed.

Following World War I, British physicians used the term *shell shock* to describe a constellation of shared physical and psychological symptoms that were found to be common among veterans. It was thought that their symptoms—fatigue, irritability, difficulty concentrating, recurrent headaches, and eventually mental breakdowns—were a manifestation of microhemorrhages of their brains caused by the shock waves of exploding shells.

Were today's physicians or psychologists to see a WWI shell-shocked Tommy, post-traumatic stress disorder (PTSD) would certainly be something they'd consider on their list of potential diagnoses. PTSD was first included in the DSM (*Diagnostic and Statistical Manual of Mental*

Disorders) in 1980, and four revisions later, it is defined as a characteristic set of symptoms seen following exposure to an extremely traumatic stressor. PTSD's formal recognition in 1980 enabled the establishment of organized research, formalized treatments, and compassionate care for millions around the globe.

So where am I going with this?

When I first opened my practice's doors in 2004, I wasn't entirely sure what to expect. People struggled with dietary organization. They didn't cook enough, they had no concept of calories, and they were skipping meals and snacks in the daytime and struggling at night. But quickly I noticed that there was a large group of patients with a common struggle, one in which the deep-rooted maladaptive emotions and behaviors fueled by dieting's seven deadly sins and traumas made thoughtful lifestyle reform an incredible challenge. These individuals shared a narrative, and while they might not have all been on the same diets or weight loss programs, they were all survivors of years—often decades—of multiple failed traumatic dieting efforts. Those failed dietary efforts and traumas, in turn, created a shared constellation of symptoms of their own—something that over time I've come to describe as "post-traumatic dieting disorder" (PTDD).

PTDD is not a trivial condition medically or psychologically. While at first blush you might be tempted to downplay its importance, medically PTDD impacts on a person's ability to safely, effectively, and sustainably lose weight; psychologically, PTDD can be devastating.

Not everyone who has suffered through traumatic diets comes down with full-blown PTDD, though almost everyone who has traumatically dieted will relate with at least some of PTDD's hallmark features.

PTDD is bred from the traumas of dieting—guilt, shame, failure, depression, despair, binge eating, and/or weight cycling. The most common constellation of symptoms include ongoing issues with:

- Feelings of ineffectiveness
- Shame
- Hopelessness

- Feeling permanently damaged
- Loss of healthy body image
- Social withdrawal
- Feeling constantly threatened by food
- Impaired relationships with others
- Change in personality

Sufferers of PTDD also often describe painful guilty feelings when eating foods that they believe are "bad," "dangerous," or simply inconsistent with what they perceive as their required weight loss diet. People with full-blown PTDD, especially in the midst of a weight loss effort, rather than face their guilt may almost phobically avoid guilt-inducing foods. This avoidance might even interfere with personal relationships and lead to marital conflict or divorce. Sufferers may also have a generalized sense of a foreshortened or bleak future, and may think themselves to be unlikely or undeserving of a career, marriage, intimacy, health, or a normal lifespan.

For too many, PTDD has its roots in childhood. It may be a consequence of being placed on restrictive diets at a very young age, or being pressured or bullied by parents or other children regarding weight. In today's climate of concern surrounding rapidly rising rates of childhood obesity, the pressure for children to diet may even come from well-intentioned authority figures. Schools have begun to distribute "BMI report cards," while pediatricians and primary care physicians are being encouraged to regularly check BMI in children. Their concerns may well be sincere and their intentions gentle, but I worry about these sorts of initiatives. The unfortunate truth is that we don't yet have an effective, reproducible, sustainable intervention that we can be confident will help these children. There's no denying that childhood obesity is a real and growing problem. Yet I don't think we're going to solve it by focusing on the children, because it's not the fault of the children; childhood obesity is a symptom of a much more insidious problem: a broken environment. Trying to fix the cause by treating just the symptom would be like responding to a flood by trying to teach everyone how to swim instead of trying to build a levee. If the flood doesn't abate, eventually even the strongest swimmers are going to fail—and this flood isn't going anywhere anytime soon.

With adults, traumatic dieting triggers would include aggressive or emotionally abusive spouses or significant others, with the abuse focused on weight loss, diet failure, physical looks, or weight as a whole. Personal triggers could include recurrent failures with prior dieting efforts, as well as suffering perceived or real weight discrimination, hatred, or scorn.

Another major traumatic dieting trigger, one that serves to spur both adults and children to destructive efforts, is the media and entertainment industries' representations and characterizations of people with obesity.

Children are regularly bombarded with weight's negative stereotypes. For example, popular movies like *Kung Fu Panda* teach children that weight is synonymous with gluttony; popular television programs like *The Simpsons* teach them it's tied to laziness; and popular books teach them that fat kids are mean and stupid, like Harry Potter's Dudley Dursley, whose weight is both a constant source of derision and scorn and an identity unto itself. While certainly the Harry Potter series includes other villains who don't happen to be obese, the author, J. K. Rowling, uses Dudley's weight to personify the worst of society's stereotypes about weight: greed, gluttony, laziness, and stupidity.

My oldest daughter first read Harry Potter at the age of seven, as did many of her peers. Despite the fact that I took the time to sit and chat with her about the way Dudley was written, I still worry about the impact he might have had on her perceptions of children with obesity. My daughter doesn't struggle with her weight, but what if she did? How do you think a markedly overweight child might react to reading about Dudley? What sort of trauma to body image, food relationship, and self-worth do you think Dudley's depiction might conjure up for them?

For adults, media and entertainment triggers are nearly constant, with editorial boards and reporters consistently portraying weight as a character flaw—Dudley's disease of lack of willpower, inactivity, and gluttonous greed. The sensationalized weight loss television shows that blanket prime time—*The Biggest Loser, Celebrity Fit Club, Heavy,* and *Extreme Makeover: Weight Loss Edition*—demonstrate anything but ease. All of these shows broadcast remarkable short-term success as a consequence of equally remarkable short-term suffering and traumatic dieting, and while these shows certainly demonstrate that there is tremendous challenge involved, at the same time they're presented in a manner that both implicitly and often explicitly tells viewers that anyone can do it. That if you just want it badly enough, you can make it happen, and unlike the contestants on the show, you might have only 50 pounds you want to lose, so clearly for you it ought to be easy. The extension, of course, is the suggestion that if you haven't made it happen despite wanting it badly enough, you're a failure. This juxtaposition between the commonly held belief that weight loss is easy, and the evidence that it is not, underlies the essential tenets of traumatic dieting: that weight is a reflection of personal weakness and failed character, and that success is predetermined by your ability to suffer and endure hardship. This may help to explain the recent and not even remotely surprising study finding that watching even a single episode of *The Biggest Loser* increased viewers' antifat biases and led them to more strongly believe that weight is easily controllable.[1]

Not only do traumatic diets not work, but these diets themselves may break people. Many individuals with PTDD share persistent symptoms of food- and weight-related anxiety or guilt that were not present before their traumatic dieting experiences. In other words, the experience of serially traumatically dieting creates new insecurities that healthy adults may not have suffered from prior to engaging in their diets. Some individuals report irritability or outbursts of anger and severe loss of self-esteem, especially following the ingestion of indulgent foods. They may snap at their spouses who bring them home a gift of chocolate, or fume at their coworkers who've decided to bring in baking. Chocolate never used to make them hate themselves, but now they may find themselves filled with self-loathing every time they allow themselves some enjoyment from a dietary indulgence. Following recurrent dieting-related trauma, PTDD sufferers may find that their body images are worse than before they began trying to lose, and as a consequence they may be less inclined to go to the beach with their families or out dancing with their friends. In more severe cases, PTDD sufferers might actively avoid all activities that reflect, amplify, or remind them of their impaired body image, which in turn may further interfere with a myriad of interpersonal relationships and lead to interpersonal conflict.

But I've left something out.

In fact, I've left out the most common and surprising feature of PTDD. I've left out the feature that back in 2004 really had me confused. It's the fact that despite all of these discouraging side effects to traumatic dieting, people keep coming back for more. It's the "Thank you sir, may I have another" approach to traumatic weight loss, and truly, the most common maladaptive behavior of patients with PTDD is their tendency to undertake recurrent and intrusive traumatic dieting efforts during which the negative symptoms are replayed again and again and again.

It's a real head-scratcher. Why would otherwise intelligent, thoughtful, and resourceful people keep putting themselves through incredibly traumatizing experiences over and over again?

I think the answer lies in the mythology of weight management. So turn to the next chapter and let's do some myth busting.

THE MYTHOLOGY OF MODERN-DAY DIETING

While there's still a great deal for us to talk about, before we go any further with how to fix things, we should discuss society's most common dieting myths that in turn perpetuate recurrent traumatic dieting, and then the one myth that rules them all and binds them all together.

MYTH: PEOPLE LACK WILLPOWER.

I hear all the time, not only from thin folks who just don't understand weight management, but even from folks who've themselves struggled for decades, that the reason people struggle is that they lack willpower, that they just can't resist temptation. Could it simply be that in just 50 short years the world has gone from a willful place to one filled with weakness?

Do you feel the same way? As I mentioned earlier, I can't agree.

Here you are: you've battled your weight possibly even since childhood, you've spent thousands of dollars and hundreds of hours on various dieting efforts, and you're blaming your own lack of willpower? As I see it as evidenced by your ongoing commitment over the years, you have incredible amounts of willpower. I'd go so far as to wager that in all likelihood, you have spent more willpower on weight management than on any other area of your life.

So is it a lack of willpower that has led to the tripling of childhood obesity rates over the course of the past 40 years? Have we suddenly raised a generation of toddlers and elementary school kids who just don't have the same stick-to-itiveness of prior generations?

Of course not.

It's not about willpower. If it were about willpower, if it were about just wanting it badly enough, the world would be skinny.

So if it's not about willpower, what is it about?

It's about change and it's about beliefs.

In terms of change, the world is a very, very different place from what it was just 50 short years ago, and there are many things that have an impact upon a person's weight.

These days, cheap calories are everywhere and everyone's telling us to eat them. Where we used to go to buy gas, there are now junk-food supermarkets. Where eating out used to be a rare treat, it's now affordable and convenient enough to be a multiple-time-a-week occurrence. Where there used to be family dinners, now there are weekly pizza nights. Where there used to be only water fountains, now there are school chocolate milk programs where each glass of the stuff contains up to double the calories of Coca-Cola, along with 20 percent more sugar. And, of course, there are newly supersized portions and tens of billions of dollars a year of food industry advertising to now contend with.

It's a different world now, and the default in this world is weight gain, and simple, brute-force willpower doesn't stand a chance.

In my opinion, dieting has proven itself to be a tremendous failure over the years. But from all angles, we are taught to believe the opposite: that diets work, it's we who fail. And beliefs matter. But couldn't it be that the fault for our never-ending dieting failures doesn't lie with us as individuals, but rather with how we approach dieting as a whole? A paradigm shift was needed for ancient astronomers to realize that the true nature of the world around them was a round, rather than a flat, earth. If we're going to make sense and success of dieting, diets need a new underlying belief, an integral part of which must include rejecting the notion that willpower is enough to see us through.

MYTH: WEIGHT AND HEALTH ARE
MUTUALLY INCLUSIVE OR EXCLUSIVE.

Another example of a mistaken belief that permeates weight loss lore is that of the unhealthy nature of weight: that a person simply cannot be considered healthy unless their weight or body mass index reaches some specific number. While there's no doubt that at the extremes of weight there's definitively attributable risk, there's also no doubt that the risks of weight as a singular measure of the presence or absence of health have been markedly overblown by both society and medicine. Some studies have even suggested that beyond the age of 65 the healthiest body weights are statistically in the medically overweight range (a body mass index between 25 and 30), and that mild degrees of medical obesity are in fact no riskier than possessing a "normal" body weight.[1] We all need to remember, patients and doctors alike, that weight doesn't exist in a vacuum, and that health has a great many variables. There are studies that demonstrate that even with moderate obesity, eating a healthful diet and exercising regularly mitigates the vast majority of risk that had been attributable to weight.[2] What I'm trying to impress upon you is that the notion that you can be healthy only if your weight is ideal, or if your body mass index ranges between 22 and 25, is flawed, and that health is far too complex to be boiled down to a number on a scale. How do you think the mistaken belief that a person can't possibly be healthy at a BMI of let's say 35 affects the person who has brought himself down from a BMI of 45? Well, I'll tell you: it leads them to feel like a failure and it might even lead them to give up entirely and regain the weight they'd lost.

So how does a person lose weight in this day and age, when it would certainly seem that the default is to gain, the environment is toxic, and the deck is conclusively stacked against us? According to the founding director of Yale University's Prevention Research Center, Dr. David Katz, it's not about developing willpower, it's about cultivating *skillpower*.

The good news is that the skills required aren't the classic triad of suffering, sacrifice, and struggle. The skills required are organization, planning, and thoughtfulness, and with those skills, it is possible not only to experience permanency with weight loss, but perhaps more important, it's possible to enjoy a normal, healthy, and friendly relationship with food. Skillpower, while it does take time to master, gets easier with time, as the more practice a person has with any particular skill, the better that person will get at it, and the more naturally it will come.

MYTH: DIETING, BY DEFINITION, MUST BE DIFFICULT.

Whoever thinks that successful weight management is about suffering doesn't understand human nature. We're not built to suffer. In fact, I'd argue that we spend the entirety of our lives trying to minimize our suffering.

Yet dieting has always classically been about some combination of undereating or overexercising, and both of those approaches invariably involve suffering.

Sure, we do things in our lives that we don't enjoy, but the only way we sustain those unenjoyable behaviors is to have no recourse—they're things we simply have to do because we have no choice. In this environment, when it comes to eating there's always recourse and always choice. Given that food is one of the most basic of human pleasures, and that in our modern dietary utopia we can buy whatever we want, whenever we want it, the notion that we're going to suffer our weights down by trying to avoid foods we enjoy is more than a little naïve.

Suffering does more damage than simply making weight management difficult to sustain. Believing oneself to be a failure as a consequence of being unable to suffer is a terrifically self-destructive and traumatic burden that in turn challenges each successive weight management effort and contemplation thereof. Truly, for weight management to last a lifetime, it can't be difficult, and going into a weight management effort believing you're going to need to suffer to succeed almost certainly guarantees that you won't.

In their book *Switch: How to Change Things When Change Is Hard*, Chip and Dan Heath explain that in order to effect long-term change, we need to improve the path we take to get to where we want to go. If the goal is long-term weight management, instead of the entrenchment of suffering—a path that is undeniably difficult—we need to focus on ways to make living with less food or fewer calories easier. Individuals who succeed in maintaining weight loss may well be more thoughtful about food and fitness, but most important, they've found a way to be more thoughtful that for them no longer qualifies as suffering. They've improved their paths.

MYTH: YOU SHOULDN'T EAT UNLESS YOU'RE HUNGRY.

If there's a more dangerous piece of dieting advice out there, I don't know what it is.

My experiences have taught me that hunger isn't your friend. Hunger is over 100 million years of evolution that has taught your body either you eat, or you die.

While scientists are slowly teasing out the neurohormonal building blocks of hunger, you needn't travel any farther than your local super-market to see how powerful they are. What happens when you go to the supermarket hungry? You buy differently—in terms of both portions and choices.

What happens when you sit down to a meal hungry?

Well, it's just like heading out to the supermarket, except that now, rather than shopping from the aisles of chips and cookies, you'll be shopping from your plate, your fridge, your freezer, your cupboards, or a menu, and guaranteed, you'll shop differently than if you sat down to that very same meal not hungry.

Remember, too, that there are many different faces to hunger. Some people will never feel true stomach-gnawing hunger, yet those very same folks may struggle with nearly insatiable cravings or emotional eating episodes.

As I mentioned earlier, I like to subdivide hunger into body or stom-ach hunger and brain hunger, with everyone experiencing a different combination of the two. But whether it's body or brain, hunger's not your friend. The body's not stupid. There's a reason we don't crave green, leafy salads when we're hungry: the body knows hunger is its cue to search for calories, and there simply aren't many calories in green, leafy salads. Hunger, whether it's from body or brain, pushes people towards carbohydrates or fats because both are important stockpiles of energy. Folks who feel they're "carb addicts" likely crave sweets when faced with body or brain hunger, while others (like me) crave salty, fatty foods like chips.

Hunger will also affect our emotional interpretation of food. Make a healthy, calorie-controlled choice when you're hungry and the choice will be bittersweet. You'll be proud that you've ordered a lower-calorie meal, but at least a small part of you will feel bitterness toward the "stupid diet" that kept you from choosing the more indulgent option you probably wanted when you read the menu. Make that very same choice sitting down to eat when not hungry, and now you'll likely be proud of your dietary discretion because you won't have had hunger telling you what you wanted.

Simply put, it's much more difficult to be happy about eating healthfully or moderately when you're hungry, and if you're not particularly happy about what you're eating, you aren't going to keep eating that way.

There's great news here. Hunger is almost always preventable, and just like going to the supermarket when you're not hungry, having actively organized your meals to prevent hunger makes it far easier to navigate calorie-controlled, healthful options.

More great news? As far as hunger prevention goes, what matters most are the frequency and protein and calorie content of your meals and snacks—and not in terms of maximums, but rather minimums. Meaning you're going to have to worry about eating enough, not about eating too much.

Hunger prevention insists you never again practice white-knuckled eating. We'll get into that in much greater detail later in the book and it will involve using time, calories, and macronutrients to shut down the body's physiologic drive towards indulgence.

MYTH: FITNESS IS MORE IMPORTANT THAN FOOD FOR WEIGHT LOSS.

Who hasn't tried the "exercise more" weight loss program? While there's likely no behavior more important to overall health than exercise, in the real world exercise doesn't drive weight loss.

Looking at real-life folks, it would seem that to lose a pound through exercise requires on the order of 70 to 90 or so hours of exercise. Of course, mathematically that makes no sense at all. Ninety hours of exercise ought to burn well over a dozen pounds' worth of calories. Whether you don't eat a calorie or burn a calorie, at the end of the day that calorie's impact on weight should be the same. Yet with the exception of controlled experimental environments, it isn't.

Where did I come up with the 70-to-90-hour number? From a couple of studies. The first one looked at the impact exercise had on Amish carriers of a known obesity gene, the FTO gene.[3] The study found that Amish FTO carriers who reported being active for 3 to 4 hours more per day than their more sedentary FTO carrier counterparts were 15 pounds lighter. That's a 72–97-hour annual difference for each and every pound—meaning that if you faithfully head to the gym for an hour a day, each and every day of the year, even if you don't take one single day off, by year's end you'll have lost only 6 pounds as a result of your exercise.

The second was a study of 196 individuals who were asked to exercise for an hour a day, six days a week, and not to make any changes to their diets.[4] The study participants were recruited out of their doctors' offices, and the researchers were looking for sedentary and unfit folks between the ages of 40 and 75. The study's exercise intervention was both home- and gym-based moderate to vigorous aerobic exercise. Study adherence was stellar, and over the course of a year, men averaged 6.16 hours of weekly exercise, and women, 4.90—that's 320 hours of exercise for the men and 254 for the women! Did they lose weight? Did literally hundreds of hours of gym time translate into movement on the scale? By the end of the year, compared with their nonexercising control group, exercising men were only 3.5 pounds lighter and women only 2.6 pounds lighter. In hours per year per pound, that works out to 91.5 hours per year to effect a 1-pound change on the scale for both men and women.

So what's going on? Shouldn't calories burned exercising have the same bottom-line impact on weight as calories not eaten? Why doesn't the math work in real life?

Because we're human.

Have you ever eaten anything "because you exercised"? An extra portion? A higher-calorie choice? A reward for your hard work? I sure have. Or have you ever been hungrier because you exercised? Me too! And once you start eating in response to your exercise, exercise's weight benefits quickly disappear.

You may also get lulled into a false sense of security by your exercise equipment, which may have a little digital display telling you how many calories you've burned exercising. I spoke with physicist and athlete Alex Hutchinson, author of *Which Comes First, Cardio or Weights? Fitness Myths, Training Truths, and Other Surprising Discoveries from the Science of Exercise,* who pointed out that the machines often grossly overestimate the calories you're actually burning. For instance, they'll assume you're running on that treadmill at 4 miles per hour rather than walking, and running burns significantly more calories because the definition of *running* dictates that you've actually got both legs off the ground in between strides, which in turn requires expending a great deal more energy. According to Hutchinson, they'll also likely include the calories you'd be burning even if you weren't exercising: "You might burn 88 calories while walking a mile, but you would have burned 36 of those calories just to stay alive for those minutes, so your net burn is just 52"—a phenomenon that's more misleading the lower your exercise intensity. Yet it's difficult to resist the urge to believe that the calories your exercise equipment reports you've burned are calories you've earned the "right" to eat.

Exercise has a tremendous impact on us psychologically and physiologically, and in regard to weight management, those impacts are both for better and for worse.

While exercise may lead us to unknowingly consume more calories as a reward for our exercise than the calories we burned exercising in the first place, there's no doubt that exercise does us many tremendously good services, and it's no myth that exercise helps us keep weight off. Exercise has a powerful impact on our mood and our sleep, and in my experience, markedly bolsters healthy living attitudes as a whole. It's likely these less tangible or indirect benefits that lead to weight management's most unfair paradox. While exercise alone is unlikely in the real world to lead to any dramatic weight loss, we know that without exercise you're far more likely to regain whatever weight you've lost. Exercise is another of those commonalities found among the National Weight Control Registry's weight loss masters. When all's said and done, most folks suggest that dietary choices are responsible for 70 to 80 percent of a person's weight, while fitness covers the remaining 20 to 30 percent.

I don't know about you, but if I had a final exam where the questions were to be weighted 70 to 80 percent in favor of one semester's material, I'm pretty sure that's the semester I'd be giving the vast majority of my study time and attention. To put this another way: it's far easier to lose weight in your kitchen than it is to lose weight in your gym.

MYTH: CHEAT DAYS MAKE DIETING EASIER.

They make sense on paper. If 86 percent of your week (six of seven days) is great, you've earned that day off. Right? What about just a meal off?

It'd still be a bad plan, but let's go through the why with some numbers. There are 21 formal meals a week. What if 95 percent of them (20 out of 21) were perfect? And I mean really perfect—homemade, from scratch, with loads of fruits and vegetables and perfect calorie control? Unfortunately, living in our modern food environment even a single "cheat" meal—a purposely indulgent, pay-no-attention, write-off meal— has the caloric potential to erase nearly an entire week of exceptionally careful choices.

Here's how.

I remember watching an episode of a weight-loss reality show. In it, contestants dined at a fancy restaurant—you know, the kind with the big plates and the small portions. The challenge involved guesstimating the calories in their ordered meals. One contestant ordered a beet salad, followed by a fish fillet plated on vegetables over a bed of what looked like couscous or brown rice. Total calories for her meal consisting of undeniably healthy ingredients? Over 2,000, and that didn't include any wine, dessert, or predinner bread.

Even if that undeniably healthy-sounding combination were your cheat meal (and chances are your cheat meal would be far more indulgent), and you also decided to have a glass of wine and share a dessert, your singular cheat meal could easily lead you to consume 2,000 more calories than you burned that day.

Putting that in some perspective: if you were aiming to lose 1.5 pounds weekly, over half your week might be spent just working off the surplus from that one single meal. If you were aiming for a 1-pound weekly loss, there went five days worth of effort. If you were just trying to maintain your weight, one indulgent cheat meal a week could lead to a 15- to 30-pound annual gain!

Have a full-fledged cheat day rather than just a cheat meal, and you can almost certainly kiss your entire week of weight loss good-bye.

But there are graver risks to cheat days than simply excess calories.

Every time you decide to "cheat," what you're doing is making it easier to do so again and again. What might start out as a weekly cheat meal may expand to a full-fledged cheat day, to weeklong cheat vacations, to stressful-time cheat months, and finally to an *all-you-can-cheat* lifestyle.

Of course, if you are feeling compelled to cheat, there are certainly other things wrong. Feeling the need to cheat means that you're living with an overly restrictive lifestyle. The belief that using food for reasons other than fuel is cheating can derail even the most sincere dieter. We don't eat purely for sustenance. Food isn't simply fuel. The roles of food, as a pleasure, a comfort, and a social pillar, are part of the very fabric of the human condition, and if it's cheating to be human, well, that's a big problem.

MYTH: SOME FOODS SIMPLY MUST BE FORBIDDEN.

At my office, I regularly write actual prescriptions for chocolate, chips, cookies, ice cream, cake, and the like.

While that might strike you as odd, the notion that a person's going to successfully and permanently avoid a particular food—especially a highly palatable, physiologically or psychologically rewarding one—is ridiculous. Inevitably, regardless of a person's dietary or weight management desires, a situation will arise where even if it's "forbidden," a danger food's going to get eaten. Whether it's a consequence of emotion, fatigue, stress, celebration, injury, or vacation, everyone knows that eventually, their forbidden foods are (at least temporarily) not always going to be forbidden.

Chocolate, ice cream, cake, chips, pizza, peanut butter, Chinese food—everyone has foods they struggle to control themselves around. For many, their strategy to deal with danger foods is to blindly restrict them—out of sight out of mind, or so the theory goes. Some people even ask their spouses to hide their most common dietary temptations. Others will freeze chocolate bars, go on black-garbage-bag-filling junk food purges, or tell their friends that they can't join them on a regular outing because of the foods available at wherever it is their friends want to go. Oftentimes, the folks who rely on forbidding food as a weight management strategy are binge eaters. These are the last folks who should live overly restrictive lifestyles as studies clearly finger overly restrictive diets as one of the primary drivers of binge eating.[5] In my clinical experience, I can also tell you I've met many a binge eater who has reported that they only began binge eating in the aftermath of their involvement in a severely restrictive diet plan or program—meaning that not only can highly restrictive diets trigger binge eating, they may also help lay the foundation of the disorder itself.

To navigate this world's dietary indulgences, a person needs to learn to switch gears from being blindly restrictive to being thoughtfully reductive. Asking questions like "Is it worth the calories?" and "What's the smallest amount of [insert forbidden food here] that I need to be happy?" can go a long way to temper forbidden food–related weight management failure.

If you're thinking to yourself, *But I can't control myself around those foods*, don't worry. I'll be teaching you how to reorganize your eating to provide you with the "willpower" you've always simply assumed you didn't have.

MYTH: CARBS ARE THE ENEMY. FATS ARE THE ENEMY.
SUGAR'S THE ENEMY. FRUCTOSE IS THE ENEMY. AND SO ON.

It seems like popular diets travel in waves. The 1990s were the low-fat decade. Next came the low-carb decade. Next maybe it'll be the low-fructose or gluten-free decade. All I know is that traumatic dieters are always given different foods on which to blame their weights.

But here's the thing. If you don't like the life you're living while you're losing, even if you lose a great deal, you're not going to keep on living that way. Given that there are only three main simplified categories of foods for diet gurus to demonize (carbohydrates, fats, or proteins), removing or vilifying one will certainly limit your dietary choices dramatically. What that means is that even if you lose a huge amount of weight by avoiding a particular food grouping, it will likely take an enormous effort to keep it out of your life forever (and even more so if you happen to enjoy that grouping's foods). Old foods return, then old calories return, and with them, old weights.

Cutting out entire food groups or categories is a dietary strategy that's like an icy cold lake. While you might be able to muster up the courage to dive in, and while you might even get numb enough while you're in to enjoy a brief frolic, once you pull yourself out, the likelihood of heading back soon thereafter for another dip's low. If you've got to numb yourself against the carbs or fats or whatever it is you're avoiding, chances are once you inevitably climb out of that icy dietary lake, you won't be rushing back in. And really, who could blame you?

The notion that there's one causal food, or category of food, that is leading society to gain weight is a dangerous one, as it leads back to the forbidden food issue. Low-carb diets, for instance, even if they're wonderful at helping you lose weight, will fail if you happen to miss the carbs you've lost enough to start eating them again. I can't tell you how many folks I've seen who have had great success on Atkins only to gain back everything they'd lost because they missed their carbs too much to sustain what was for them an overly restrictive diet.

That's not to say that modifying the building blocks of a diet can't help. It's just that there's no one-size-fits-all magic formula. Of course, if you don't make any changes to your style of eating, you're not likely going to lose weight, but what I aim to do is to teach you how to use food to control it, rather than let food control you. At the end of the day, regardless of what changes you make to your diet, the secret to maintaining your losses is to honestly enjoy what you're eating, and of course, to consume fewer calories than you used to. If low-carb or low-fat works for you to the point where you feel confident that you can keep living that way for the rest of your life, I'd never tell you to stop.

MYTH: YOU'RE NOT LOSING WEIGHT BECAUSE YOU'RE BUILDING MUSCLE.

Have you ever told yourself that? You'd been working out for weeks, possibly even months, in a gym, and the scale wasn't budging. Either you told yourself, or your trainer told you, that the reason the scale wasn't moving was because you were building muscle and that muscle weighs more than fat. If only muscle were that easy to build. While it's true that during the first few weeks of weight training your body might see a slight increase in water weight, consequent to increased glycogen storage, without the help of dangerous and illegal anabolic steroids, building muscle is truly a full-time job. It takes dozens if not hundreds of hours of consistency in the gym to effectively build pounds and pounds of muscle—and here I'm not talking about gentle walks on the treadmill and a BodyPump class, I'm talking about real weight lifting. More important, though, there's nothing that would stop your body from simultaneously losing fat and building muscle. If you're eating fewer calories than you burn, providing your body with sufficient nutritional building blocks to build muscle, and putting your time in at the gym, you'll be losing fat and building muscle at the same time. You'll also be losing weight. At the end of the day, if you're not losing weight, the laws of thermodynamics dictate you're eating as many calories as you're burning.

The myth that we're not losing weight because we're building muscle, when coupled with the myth that exercise burns huge numbers of calories, seems somewhat counterintuitive. Yet many of us cling to both of those beliefs. Perhaps the myth of muscle weight serves to help explain the intuitive but erroneous belief that exercise burns tremendous numbers of calories?

Of course, folks who think they can simply burn off an evening of indulgences through exercise will undoubtedly be disappointed by their scales over time. Even folks who are trying to work off only the occasional treat, unless they truly appreciate the calories involved in both their food and fitness, may find themselves scratching their heads. Putting treats into some perspective: let's say your once-weekly hard-earned indulgence is a lazy Sunday morning skim milk latte and blueberry scone at Starbucks. To burn that off will take a 180-pound person nearly 90 minutes of walking. If that person gets discouraged because the addition of 90 minutes of weekly walking doesn't seem to be getting them anywhere, in the beginning they may decide that they're not losing weight because they're building muscle. But eventually, with enough time and disappointment, they might decide that they're simply incapable of weight loss. Despite having started their weekly walking program with the intention of healthier living, being disappointed by a lack of exercise-mediated weight loss might lead them to abandon it altogether.

Too bad, too, because even in the absence of weight change, there's probably nothing that a person can do that would be more beneficial to their health than regular exercise.

MYTH: IF YOU KNOW YOU'RE GOING TO HAVE A HIGH CALORIE NIGHT, YOU BETTER MAKE SURE YOU SKIMP ALL DAY.

This myth is incredibly pervasive, and incredibly destructive.

We've already discussed the impact of hunger on choice. So what happens if you're having a big meal out that you show up for hungry because you've been "saving" up your calories for it? You'll probably say hello to the bread basket, order an appetizer, finish your main course, and ask to see the dessert menu. The appetizer alone will likely contain more calories than you've "saved" all day long. That's not helpful math for your weight management effort. Skipping 500 daytime calories can easily lead you to consume 1,500 calories you'd otherwise have been able to proudly, happily, and easily avoid.

So yes, you may have been able to "save" a few hundred calories by being a stingy eater all day long, but you're going to pay dearly at night.

Instead of starving yourself all day in order to stuff yourself all night, the real trick is to be thoughtful and organized with your eating throughout the day. Show up to your festive or social meal not hungry, and you'll give yourself the ability to thoughtfully navigate the table. Suddenly, you won't need your own appetizer, you'll easily be able to skip the bread, and you might not want to finish your main course. Dessert? Maybe, but certainly not a given and probably not the whole thing. In fact, if you navigate the table thoughtfully, by arriving not hungry, you might easily avoid an entire day's worth of hunger-driven calories.

MYTH: THERE'S WEIGHT LOSS IN THAT THERE BOTTLE.

If only there were a natural weight loss product that made a remarkable difference. Suffice it to say that if there were a product, pill, or potion that had a remarkable, safe, and reproducible impact on weight, I'd be doing something else with my medical degree.

While there is no shortage of products claiming they'll help you to lose weight, there's a complete lack of scientific studies to back up their claims. If the study's been done, the fact that it's not on my desk, that there aren't drug or nutraceutical company representatives beating down my and my colleagues' doors study in hand, would suggest that the outcomes of the study weren't particularly remarkable.

In 2004, two professors of complementary medicine, Max Pittler and Edzard Ernst, published a systematic review of the most commonly touted natural weight loss aids and products.[6] They looked at chitosan, chromium picolinate, *Ephedra sinica*, *Garcinia cambogia*, glucomannan, guar gum, hydroxy-methylbutyrate, plantago psyllium, pyruvate, yerba maté, and yohimbe. Their conclusion was very straightforward: "The evidence for most dietary supplements as aids in reducing body weight is not convincing. None of the reviewed dietary supplements can be recommended for over-the-counter use."

For both drug and nutraceutical companies, a safe and effective weight management product is their holy grail, and like the grail, it has yet to be found.

MYTH: THE LAST 10 POUNDS ARE THE HARDEST.

I can't tell you how many times I've heard that statement. There are even television shows and boot camps dedicated to those "last" 10 pounds.

What does that mean—*last*? For most people, it means the last 10 pounds to go before getting to a preset number goal.

But if you have to try that much harder to lose them, they're probably not staying off; if those 10 pounds require effort above and beyond what you're comfortable living with happily ever after, their loss will last only as long as you sustain your now superhuman efforts.

I prefer to swap adjectives. Instead of those pounds being the "hardest," I think it's fair to say that they'll be the "slowest," because as a person gets smaller, for a variety of reasons, they literally burn fewer calories. Therefore, the closer you get to your eventual final weight resting place, the slower those pounds will come off.

"Harder" suggests nonsustainable, and whatever interventions, diets, exercises, etc. you employ to lose the weight—if you don't sustain them, your weight will undoubtedly return, and so will those "last 10 pounds."

They also might not be the *only* 10, since for many folks, regain is so demoralizing that they often abandon all of their weight-related interventions, so not only will those "last" 10 come back, eventually the "first" 10 will, too.

THE ONE MYTH THAT RULES THEM ALL: OUR WEIGHTS SHOULD ALL BE "IDEAL."

In every other area of life, people are comfortable with their personal bests as wonderful goals. Why is it that with weight people strive to be "ideal," often at the expense of a liveable life?

"Ideal" is quite the lofty goal. The dictionary definition is "absolute perfection," and it ignores the simple truth that with every human characteristic there's a wide range of what could and should be considered normal.

Many people trying to lose weight seem to be focused on their body fat percentages, their "ideal" weights, their body mass indices, their waist circumferences, or their waist-to-hip ratios—the weights and measures that a table, a calculator, a public health official, or an allied health professional says they ought to possess as a function of their height, age, and sex.

Of course, all of these idealized weights and values ignore reality. Idealizing weights and body mass indices also ignores the fact that weights will vary across races, sexes, and ages, and are affected by things like frame size and musculature. For instance, over half of the NFL would be considered "obese" if we used BMI to judge them.[7]

The fact is, our weights are influenced by a huge number of factors, some within our control and some beyond it. Genetics, coexisting medical conditions, required medications, how long and stressful your workday is, how well you sleep, how old you are, how old your children are, whether your job requires you to take clients out to restaurants, whether you enjoy exercise, what types of foods you grew up on—there is no shortage of variables that have very real bearings on our weights.

Ultimately, ideal weights don't matter in the face of reality, and reality in turn will affect what I'll refer to as your "best" weight.

To help illustrate what I mean, let's stop for a minute and talk about running and the Boston Marathon.

Two years ago I turned 40. That bought me an extra five-minute cushion for my Boston Marathon qualifying time. But here's the thing: I'm an incredibly slow runner, and I've yet to run a marathon. That said, I'd like to run one, and I figure a realistic time for me, knowing my running history and inherent speed, will likely be somewhere around the 4:30 mark.

But let's say I get it in my head that my goal isn't just to run a marathon and try my best, but rather my goal is to run a marathon and qualify for Boston. The way I see it, there are only two possible outcomes:

1. I qualify.
2. I don't.

Exploring outcome number one, I'm quite sure qualifying wouldn't come easy for me given I'm anything but a natural-born runner. In a best-case scenario, it would likely involve me painfully training for nearly a year. I'd have to neglect my family, abandon my patients, and hurt all the time from the insane amount of running I'd need to be doing.

Here's something else I'm pretty sure of. Even if I did qualify for Boston after crazy amounts of training, I'm certain that when I finally ran Boston, my time would be slower than my qualifying run. Why? Because why would I sustain a level of training that very negatively impacted upon my quality of life if I'd already achieved my goal of qualifying?

Exploring outcome number two, if after quality-of-life-reducing amounts of training for a year I didn't come anywhere near qualifying, chances are I'd stop training altogether, because there would be no point of continuing to try if my goal was qualifying for Boston and I came up way short after all of that incredibly hard work.

I think you probably see where I'm going with this.

Setting a massive, idealized, numerical weight loss goal simply isn't wise. If you have to suffer to get there, you probably won't stay there. And if you suffer only to fall short, you'll probably stop your suffering, too.

For me, my running goal will simply be running. Yes, a marathon is actually on my bucket list, but if every time I start running distances I begin to hurt too much, or simply hate it, chances are I'll just take it off my list. Really, at the end of the day, my running goal is to be able to look back upon my training and feel like I did my best. Not the best I could tolerate, but the best I could enjoy.

That's not so strange. Generally, we accept our personal bests as great at most everything, and if I feel I tried my best, I'll be all right with that.

What's truly strange is that when it comes to weight, people tend not to want to accept their personal bests as great. Somehow, when it comes to weight, everyone seems to think the goal isn't their best, but rather it's to qualify for the Boston Marathon of weight loss—reaching their so-called ideal weight, even when it's possible that so-called ideal was foisted on them by their doctor or trainer, some chart in a book, an Internet calculator, or some cockamamie television show.

Well, I'm here to tell you that your best is great, and whatever weight you reach when you're living the healthiest life you enjoy, that's your "best" weight. That said, I'm guessing too, there's probably room for your life to be healthier and still enjoyable.

So if you qualify for Boston, well, that's a heady bonus, but your real goal? Your real goal is just to enjoy your running—pace and time notwithstanding.

Only three people medal in any given race. What a shame it would be if no one ran races for fear of not medaling. When it comes to weight loss, not everyone is going to medal, and that's okay. It's far more important to enjoy the life you're living while you're losing than it is to make weight loss the sole focus of your life—because doing that, once you cross that finish line, you're liable to stop trying.

Your weight loss goal shouldn't be a number; it should be whatever weight you reach while living the healthiest life you honestly enjoy. That's your "best" weight, your personal best, and while there will be others who are likely better at losing than you, they don't matter.

The healthiest life you can enjoy is very different than the healthiest life you can tolerate.

You might think that's easier said than done.

I've got good news for you. I think you can find that life in just 10 short days. Ten days to effectively press the Reset button on perhaps even decades of traumatic dieting. And I'm going to show you how.

The 10-Day Reset

What if in 10 days you could change your relationship with food forever? What if in 10 days you learned how to "eat just one"? What if in 10 days you controlled food, rather than letting food control you? What if in 10 days you could not only be in control, but also losing weight? What if in 10 days food, even so-called danger food, could be your friend? What if in 10 days your experiences led you to feel—perhaps for the first time in decades—that there was hope?

Is there anything you couldn't put up with for just 10 days?

Looking back on your traumatic diets over the years, think of what you've endured. Soup diets? Cleanses? White-knuckle cravings? Stomach-gnawing hunger? Meal replacement shakes? Endless grilled boneless, skinless chicken breasts on salads? I'd bet for many, the list is lengthy.

But what if 10 days was enough for you to press the Reset button on your whole relationship with food and your life? If in 10 days, you learned how to use food in a manner that left you with the ability to stay in thoughtful control without a fight? If in 10 days you weren't white-knuckling your way past your cupboards in the evening? If in 10 days you could still eat out with your friends? If in 10 days dietary indulgences were allowed but didn't risk excess? If in 10 days your understanding and your intentions matched your choices and your actions? If in just 10 days you were in control, because after all, if you're aiming to make a permanent dent in weight, isn't control the key?

What I'm going to present to you is a 10-Day Reset plan, 10 days during which, if you follow my directions, you'll realize that the way you and the past 150 years of diet books have been approaching your weight, your food, and your fitness, far from being helpful, were almost certainly harmful. Ten days to set you up with a basic pattern than unlike traditional "dieting" can be happily and healthfully followed for life.

I know—it sounds too good to be true. And I'm often the guy quoted in the media as saying "If it sounds too good to be true, it probably is."

What I'm promising you isn't a way to drop four pants sizes in less than two weeks, or a way to get your cholesterol levels into a healthier range overnight; the 10-Day Reset is about lifting the guilt, the fear, and the traumas of the past off of your shoulders and giving you a brand-new relationship with your body, your weight, and your health. But even if you're skeptical—and given what many traumatic dieters have been through, I certainly couldn't blame you for skepticism—it's just 10 days. Do you really have anything to lose?

Over the course of the next 10 days, you're going to train yourself that a healthy lifestyle isn't an icy cold lake. You'll learn how to use food to control it, rather than letting it control you. You'll shut down your most powerful cravings, make friends with the all-powerful scale, learn how to indulge in previously forbidden foods, and eat out in a restaurant. Most important, you'll hit the Reset button that ultimately will allow you to break free of traumatic dieting's restrictive restraints.

Each day will focus on developing a new skill set, and then each successive day will build off your previous day's success.

Don't be in a hurry. The "hurry up and lose" attitude is one of reality television, not actual reality, and just as with everything valuable in life, success takes time and skills take practice. Ten days from now, you'll have the courage and the confidence for your next 10 days, and so on, and so forth. After all, this is about cultivating and crafting a healthy relationship with food—one that's going to last you the rest of your life. And because we're talking about the rest of your life, and not just the few months before swimsuit season, there's no need to be in a rush.

Resist the urge to jump ahead and compact multiple Reset days into one. Even if you think *This day sounds easy, I'm going to skip ahead*, take it one day at a time. Do a great and thoughtful job with each and every day. And remember that timing matters. Starting your 10-Day Reset right before a major life event isn't going to stack your deck in your favor. You need a 10-day stretch when you'll be comfortable dedicating at least 30 minutes a day to this effort. Those 30 minutes aren't going to be spent killing yourself in a gym or sparring with your cupboards; they will be spent thinking, planning, organizing, and reflecting. I also don't want you overdoing it. Taking a flying leap at change is the sort of thing that can land you on your face. I'd rather you took small steps and got somewhere than take a flying leap only to reaffirm the fact that people can't fly.

While there will still be a lifetime ahead of you, in just 10 short days you will prove to yourself that a healthy relationship with food is not only possible—it's easier than you ever imagined. By the end of Day 10 you'll have learned that success is determined not through suffering and sacrifice, but rather through organization and empowerment.

Ten days to set you free from your forged-in-the-caves-of-evolution quest for calories, from society's dieting mythology, and from using calories for judgment. By reorganizing the timing of your meals and snacks and ensuring you eat enough calories and protein (no upper limits here, just lower limits), you'll empower yourself with *physiologic freedom* by turning down physiologic hunger; with *psychological freedom* by learning new ways to think about healthy living and reframing diet-centricity; and with *caloric freedom* by learning to use calories for guidance, and never for judgment.

Ultimately, by the end of Day 10 you'll have laid the foundation of behaviors and thinking that will change your relationship with food forever and stop your vicious cycle of traumatic dieting. Reset gets easier with time, as Reset is based on organization and thinking, rather than surrender and starvation. There are no foods you can't eat and no caloric glass ceilings you can't crash. There's also no formal "diet," so consequently you can employ these strategies to manage *any* approach to weight control, as long as it's an approach you honestly enjoy and can truly see yourself living with for the rest of your life.

There is absolutely no reason you can't do this. There's nothing I'll be asking you to do that isn't easily doable for everyone, let alone for someone who may well have had the willpower to lose weight on programs built on suffering. If you can suffer through traditional and traumatic diets, this Reset should be a walk in the park. The whole purpose of your Reset is to provide you with a means to succeed without suffering.

So think of Reset as a 10-day science experiment, with you as the test subject. Ten days to hit the Reset button on a lifetime of traumatic diets and diet-centric thinking. Ten days to clear out cobwebs, beat rugs, and sweep up dust. Ten days to illuminate the path to the end of traumatic dieting.

Each day of Reset begins with its own start-of-day and end-of-day checklist. Be honest about them, and if you've not been able to check off each item, hang back and repeat a day. Healthy living, which necessitates a healthy and realistic relationship with food, is a lifelong affair; time is something you have plenty of. But I know you're probably eager to see what's planned, so here are your next 10 days in brief.

DAY 1: GEAR UP

Do you go on trips without packing your bags first? Day 1 is meant for you to gather together the tools you're going to need to embark on this new journey, as well as to start cultivating your new nontraumatic life-style.

DAY 2: DIARIZE

If you ask a scientist what is the most important contributor to their ex-periment's success, bar none, they're going to say "good data." On Day 2 you're going to learn not only how to keep good data, but how to do so without trauma. Good data are there for guidance, not for judgment, and by learning to track and utilize things like your DDD score (day's degree of difficulty), you're going to learn how to become the scientist who puts you back in control of food, rather than have food continue to control you. When you're good at it, your diary will take you no more than five minutes a day of effort—five minutes that, if you're trying to lose weight, have been clinically proven to double your losses.

DAY 3: BANISH HUNGER

Hunger wins. You might be the smartest, most motivated person on the planet, but if you're regularly hungry, you're going to struggle. Starting on Day 3, you're going to learn how to organize meal and snack timing, calories, and protein to turn off stomach-growling hunger, along with "I just need a taste of that" cravings and everything in between.

DAY 4: COOK

If you want to be in control of food, you need to know what you're putting into your own body. Day 4 is about making friends with your kitchen, as you're far more likely to cultivate a healthy life and weight with the help of your kitchen than you would with the help of your gym. The good news is, it definitely doesn't need to be gourmet, nor does it need to be time or labor intensive.

DAY 5: THINK

After possibly decades of traumatic diets, chances are you're incredibly hard on yourself when it comes to healthy living. Day 5 is about truly embracing your personal best and learning how to stop beating yourself up when things go awry, and instead learning the two-step approach that will allow you to make the best of any situation.

DAY 6: EXERCISE

Exercise is the best medicine ever created, but it doesn't need to involve sweat-bursting-out-of-your-brow or want-to-throw-up intensity. In fact, it doesn't even require a gym. On Day 6 you're going to learn my eight-word fitness manifesto, that consistency is worlds more important than sweat and intensity, and how to determine your "toothbrush level" of fitness.

DAY 7: INDULGE

Simply put, real life includes chocolate (and chips, ice cream, and so many other delicious but not built for health or weight foods), and on Day 7 you're going to learn a simple two-step process to thoughtfully handle one of life's most seminal pleasures—indulgent foods.

DAY 8: EAT OUT

If you can't join your best friends for dinner, or go out to celebrate your birthday or a promotion, what kind of life would you be living? On Day 8 you're going to learn the dead-simple if counterintuitive strategy of pre-eating, along with a grab bag of easy-to-employ strategies designed to make your meals out a controllable and pleasurable breeze.

DAY 9: SET GOALS

Numbers on scales aren't good goals. Neither are clothing sizes or body fat percentages. On Day 9 you're going to learn how to set actually useful goals, goals that in turn might lead you to achieving those number goals you'd set in your traumatic dieting past.

DAY 10: TROUBLESHOOT AND MOVE FORWARD

You've got the rest of your life ahead of you, and no doubt it's not going to be a straight line. On Day 10 you're going to learn how to navigate some of the most common roadblocks and hurdles to lifelong success, along with my 10 cardinal rules designed to dust you off and prop you back up should life throw you a hard curve.

You absolutely CAN do this. I want to take just a moment and talk about the most important thing you're going to need, and it's not something you can buy—it's patience.

If there were a quick, easy, and permanent weight loss solution, the world would be skinny. This isn't going to be a rapid weight loss program, and from Day 1 I need you to stop and consider the fact that your weight today, tomorrow, and even next week isn't what matters most. What matters most, if you're concerned about your weight, is your weight a year or two from now. If you're in a big hurry, you're reading the wrong book. But I'll tell you—and I'm guessing at least rationally and intellectually you already know this—the only way to lose weight in a hurry is by doing something nonsustainable: undereating, overexercising, or both. And the fact remains, if fast were permanent, I'd be working in an emergency room somewhere.

What you're trying to do is gain a new skill set, and of course developing new skills takes time. And, yes, you might be able to picture in your mind's eye what your healthier lifestyle ought to look like, but just because you can picture what you think it ought to look like doesn't mean you'll be able to live it automatically or effortlessly. Take martial arts, for instance. I'd bet you can picture a jumping, spinning, hook kick in your mind's eye, too, but you'd never expect that knowing what it might look like would afford you the ability to do one. Instead, if you wanted to learn how, you'd start with the basics, and slowly but surely improve. The same can be said to be true with healthy living, and just like you'd never expect to earn a black belt in 10 days, don't beat yourself up for still being a white belt here.

"HOW MUCH WEIGHT WILL I LOSE?"

So how much will you lose these 10 days, and how much will you lose in total if you stick with this plan?

I have no idea. There's actually no way of knowing. I'm not suggesting you won't lose every last ounce that you'd like, but I'm also not suggesting that you will. What do I mean? Let's say you'd like to lose 70 pounds. If you ask me, "Can I lose 70 pounds?" I'll answer "Yes." It's just that "Can I lose 70 pounds" isn't a helpful or fair question. Of course, you can lose 70 pounds—you could probably lose even more than that if you really put your mind to it. Suffering and sacrifice can probably get you to any weight you want. It's just that suffering and sacrificing your way down means you're most assuredly going to go back up.

A better question to ask would be, "Can I lose 70 pounds living a life I honestly enjoy?" Now, that's a very different question, isn't it? Because really, if you lose 70 pounds living a life you enjoy, there's a great chance that you'll never gain it back again, because if you enjoyed the life you were living while you lost, there'd be no reason to stop living it once you stopped losing.

And that brings me to the best question you could possibly ask. It takes numbers out of the picture entirely and is simply: "What's the healthiest life I can honestly enjoy?" Because even if you lost only half as much as you wanted, taking 10 times longer than you expected, never gaining anything you lost back would be far more valuable than losing every last ounce doing something too severe to sustain and then gaining all of those ounces back again. After all—and I realize I'm a bit of a broken record here—regardless of the number staring back at you on the scale, if you can't happily eat less, you probably won't eat less, and if you can't happily exercise more, you won't exercise more. Therefore, whatever weight you reach when you're living the healthiest life you can enjoy, that's your *best* weight—and whatever that weight may be, it's fantastic!

You simply can't do better than your best, and your best is always great. ◉

Remember that unless you like the life you're living while you're losing, even if you lose a lot you're almost certainly going to gain it back. Because if you don't like the life you're living while you're losing, eventually you're going to find yourself going back to the life you were living before you lost. That life will bring back all of your old foods and habits, and with them, all of your old calories. Those old calories in turn will bring back all of your old weight. To put it another way: if you lose weight through suffering, when you get sick of suffering and revert back to your old lifestyle, your old weight will return with it.

Yes, it's going to take some effort, but unlike your traumatic dieting experiences, the effort required is going to involve planning, organizing, and thinking, not suffering, sacrificing, and restricting. What you need to do to improve your health may not in and of itself be complicated, but finding the time and skill to do so in this current obesogenic environment undoubtedly is. Cultivating these skills is about living a longer, better, more functionally independent, literally less painful life. It's about improving the health of your family and perhaps becoming less reliant on medications. It's about becoming friends with food and learning how to use it for both comfort and celebration, and doing so thoughtfully and in control. It's about allowing yourself to be imperfect and embracing the fact that your needs are important.

Like anything valuable in life—education, marriage, parenthood, work—you'll get out what you put in, so take your time and try it all. You've got nothing to lose and freedom from a lifetime of traumatic dieting to gain.

And if you're ready—let's go!

DAY 1: GEAR UP!

Camping wouldn't be much fun without a tent and some matches. While you might be excited to rush into things, setting out on an expedition without ensuring you're properly outfitted is a recipe for disaster. Before you go about resetting years or even decades of traumatic dieting, in order to maximize your chance of success there are a few things you'll need to have on hand. You might want to start Day 1 on a Saturday because you might well need to do some basic shopping, and having two days to get yourself organized, even if it's called "Day 1," may be helpful.

So what will you need?

SCALES AND OTHER MEASURING TOOLS

Guessing doesn't work. Our eyes, honed by hundreds of millions of years of evolution, are designed to catch moving objects, not to weigh them. Consequently, you're going to need scales—one for you, and one for food.

The "for you" scale doesn't need to agree with anyone else's scale, but it does need to agree with itself; it doesn't matter if your scale and your doctor's or your gym's scales disagree with each other, but you must trust your home scale to give you an accurate reading in order to objectively track any trends in your weight.

You know you've got a good scale if when you step on it five times in a row, it gives you pretty much the same number each and every time. Now, I don't want you weighing yourself multiple times a day, or even daily for that matter. What I recommend is weighing yourself only twice in this first 10-day journey. Once today and once the morning of Day 10, as day-to-day weight fluctuations are fairly normal and we're not looking for any rapid change. I would hate it if a scale reflecting a bit of constipation or water retention, with a slight gain, distracted you from what you're trying to accomplish.

The other scale you should pick up is for food, and this one should be digital. Those old-school basket scales with springs? They're a huge pain, as food doesn't always fit well in them, they need to get washed between weighs, and over time they become inaccurate because they work by means of a spring. Digital scales, on the other hand, are invaluable and their zero button (sometimes also called a "tare" button) helps to make weighing foods a task that takes just an extra few seconds.

PRO TIP

Most digital food scales with zero buttons zero as they're turned on— which means if you place your plate on the scale and *then* turn it on, the scale's automatic zeroing will allow you to start measuring your portions even as you plate them. ⊙

You can find digital kitchen scales in virtually any big-box store, and a basic model shouldn't cost you more than $30.

You'll also need measuring spoons and cups. Given how inexpensive the spoons and cups are, consider owning at least two complete sets so that if one's in the dishwasher, you'll have another set on hand. Your local dollar-style store is your best bet for a cheap buy here.

A JOURNAL

There's nothing more powerful than knowledge, but you can't truly gain knowledge without good data. I'm sure you'll agree; the more information you have before you make any decision in life, the better that decision will be. Your food diary is all about information. What it's not about is judgment.

I'll get into the nitty-gritty of keeping a nonjudgmental food diary on Day 2, but when you're out shopping for one I want you to appreciate that just like an actual diary, it'll record your highs and your lows. While certainly you're welcome to purchase a formal, task-oriented food diary (you can find these in bookstores and office supply stores), some may prefer a beautiful writing journal, while others may want to download a food diarizing app for their smartphone, or keep it on a spreadsheet, or enter information into an online food tracker.

If you choose the app route, my personal favorites are MyNetDiary and MyFitnessPal. Unlike virtually every other app I've looked at, MyNetDiary allows you to track the timing of your meals and snacks, while MyFitnessPal has perhaps an easier-to-use interface and a terrific social network built in. Both produce complementary apps for iPhones, iPads, BlackBerries, and Android OS, which means you can enter information by way of your smartphone when you're out and about, and via your computer when you're at your desk. My hope, too, is that by the time this book is published, I'll have my own Diet Fix Reset app, which in turn will work in concert with this book.

Apps are great for folks who might be too shy to record in public, as by using smartphones, it'll just look like you're texting someone or sending an e-mail, and having not missed a day for nearly three years now, I can tell you that when you're good at it (which takes a few weeks), it'll take a grand total of 2 to 5 minutes a day to use.

FOOD

You don't need to buy 10 days' worth of groceries today, but you do need to commit to going grocery shopping. Take a look at your weekly schedule and figure out at least one, if not two, logical food shopping slots, and actually pen or type them into your formal schedule. Getting Reset involves using food to minimize hunger, cravings, and compulsive eating. If you're concerned about your weight, you should know that the lion's share of your weight is a consequence of caloric intake, not caloric output; if you don't have food on hand, even the greatest and noblest of dietary intentions will fall by the wayside.

The First Shopping Cart of the Rest of Your Life

I'll cover food and nutrition more specifically in this book's next section. But for now, here is some basic guidance and a few suggestions that take into account that some carbohydrates, fats, and proteins are healthier and more helpful than others.

FOOD WITH A CAPITAL F

First things first. There are two kinds of food these days—I call them Capital-F Food and lowercase-f food.

Capital-F Food is actual food. Capital-F Food is sold around the perimeter of your supermarket. It includes fresh fruits and vegetables, fresh meats and fish, real nuts, legumes, and grains. It doesn't come in a bag or a box, and if it does, it's usually minimally processed with ingredients you're familiar with.

Lowercase-f food is what you want to try to minimize. Lowercase-f food is the heavily processed stuff. It's the stuff that has dozens of ingredients, many of which you can't pronounce. While lowercase-f food often tastes great, nutritionally it's often full of diabetes-inducing refined grains, blood pressure–raising sodium, and calorie-boosting sugars and fats. Unfortunately, it's the lowercase-f foods that make up the bulk of our supermarket's selections, and many of them come in packages that explicitly set out to convince you that their contents are healthy, good-for-you choices— think granola bars that tout their whole grains, "fruit" snacks "made with real fruit," and breakfast cereals that, along with 3 teaspoons of sugar in a bowl, "are a source of 9 essential nutrients." Basically, if a box tries to convince you its contents are healthy, there's a great chance that they're not.

Your shopping cart isn't meant to be a source of shame. I don't want you to think that lowercase-f foods are not allowed. I eat lowercase-f foods, too; they're a part of our world and to simply avoid them is a blind ▶

restriction that's likely not sustainable. Personally, I try to eat the smallest amount of lowercase-f food that I need in my life to be happy and satisfied. Sometimes I'll eat them out of necessity because there aren't any other options, sometimes because of convenience, and sometimes it'll be because like everyone else, I like junky foods, too.

It's important to note that reducing lowercase-f foods in your life is something that's likely going to take time. If you're not used to regular cooking with Capital-F Foods, don't worry about becoming a convert overnight. Instead try to bring in new meals slowly. As you find healthier alternatives, try to bump one of your least healthy lowercase-f food options off your cooking rotation. ◉

So what's going into your cart?

Your goal is to slowly improve the quality of your diet, not to miraculously transform into someone or something that you're not. All of our carts, mine included, could likely include healthier choices. The important thing is that the choices we made we actually thought about. Here are some considerations you might want to take into account as you're shopping and picking up those three simplified categories of food: proteins, fats, and carbohydrates.

Proteins

Proteins are actually found most everywhere. Even grains and vegetables contain protein. But if you're not a vegetarian or a vegan, chances are the bulk of your dietary protein is going to come from animal sources. Whether it's actual cuts of meat or seafood, or products made from the milk of various animals (cheeses, yogurts, etc.), those are most likely going to be your go-to sources. If you *are* a vegetarian or a vegan, chances are the bulk of your protein is going to come from pulses (beans, lentils, peas, chickpeas), nuts, and—important to single out—soy-based products (tofu, many mock meats, etc.).

Starting on Day 3 I'll be recommending that you consume protein with every meal and snack, so you'll want to have some breakfast proteins (eggs, dairy products, perhaps some protein-fortified cereal), snack proteins (nuts, single-serving yogurts or cheeses, protein bars), and lunch/dinner proteins (meats, fish, soy products, beans, etc.). Please buy solid sources if you can. Liquid protein sources (dairy and nondairy milks, meal replacement shakes, drinkable yogurts, etc.) don't leave you feeling as full as solids do so, for instance, a glass of milk isn't going to cut it as a stand-alone protein.

Fats

Fats have gotten a really bad rap over the years. While for decades we've been taught that the saturated fats found in meats and butters were basically heart attacks waiting to happen, the past few years of research have fairly conclusively exonerated fat from being risky to your heart health (excepting of course the risk of non-naturally occurring trans fats).[1] So please don't be taken advantage of by "low-fat" food labeling and go out of your way to always eat "lean." Sure, fat has more calories per gram than carbohydrates or proteins, and I definitely care about calories, but sacrificing flavor and eating pleasure by trying to eat the low-fat versions of everything isn't necessary.

Trans-fat, on the other hand, has no place in your diet. Simply put: it's a toxin unsafe in any amount and should be avoided. Baked goods are the most common place to find artificially created trans-fats, as they help to prolong shelf life. Food labeling laws are sneaky, too, in that products that contain small amounts of trans-fats are allowed to say that they contain zero, so make sure you read the label. If it says "partially hydrogenated" anything, put it back on the shelf. There are naturally occurring trans-fats in ruminants (animals that chew their cud) and their related products (primarily dairy), but the evidence would suggest you need not worry too much about those.

Carbohydrates

First off, you don't have to have them. That doesn't mean I'm telling you to go on a low-carb diet. Rather, the evidence base to date suggests that low-carb diets are safe. So if you've enjoyed low-carb living in the past, but stopped because you were worried it wasn't good for you, feel free to consider going back to a low-carb lifestyle.

That said, there are plenty of folks who have lost weight and maintained those losses eating plenty of carbohydrates. Eating bread and starches will most certainly not doom you to long-term failure.

Refined carbohydrates are the carbohydrates you want to try to minimize. They're the white stuff and the instant stuff. White sugars, white flours, white rice, and pretty much anything with the word *instant* on it (for instance, instant oatmeal). The word *refined* has to do with the processing, which in turn strips off the carbs' protective fibrous sheaths and allows your body easy access to their building block sugars; you can almost think of them as *prechewed*. These are the carbohydrates that are most likely linked to chronic disease. There have even been studies that suggest eating calorically equal amounts of refined versus whole carbohydrates ultimately allows the body to extract more calories from the refined. Consumption of refined carbs may have a larger impact on the body's insulin response, and they aren't as satiating as their slower-to-digest healthier cousins, the whole. This means that they may have a double whammy effect on weight management.

Whole carbohydrates aren't artificially processed. You can find these by ensuring the words *whole grain* come before the word *flour*, and by avoiding anything that can be cooked in an instant. Brown rice, whole grain flours, ancient whole grains like quinoa and bulgur—these are the better choices. In fact, there's very strong evidence to suggest diets higher in whole grains reduce a person's risk of developing type 2 diabetes.

While I'm not suggesting you immediately banish all that's white from your home, do take some time and experiment with some whole options. Perhaps over time, you can rid your home of the white stuff.

Fruits and vegetables also fall into the carbohydrate catchall. For the most part, they're all wonderful. The only possible exception is the potato: Dr. Walter Willett, Harvard's chair in nutrition since 1991 and the world's second-most-cited scientist in history, once suggested that consuming one was akin to spooning pure white table sugar into your mouth.[2]

That said, I do have one real caution on which fruits to buy. It stems from the fact that there is no such thing as a juice tree. Juice is not a fruit. Per drop, juice has the same amount or more of both sugar and calories when compared with sugared soda. If you agree that adding vitamins and minerals to Coca-Cola wouldn't make it a healthy choice, then you should probably reconsider that morning glass of orange juice, as that's all it really is—flat soda pop with vitamins, from which the processing has removed the vast majority of the fruit's actual nutrition. Similarly, those fruit roll-ups, gummies, and leathers—candy with a smidgen of vitamins—are definitely not fruit.

GO EASY ON THE LIQUIDS

It's not just juice that has us drinking on the pounds, it's the cream in our coffees, the milk with our cookies and our nightcaps after long days of work. Liquid calories deserve special mention, as unlike their solid counterparts, liquid calories aren't filling—meaning we don't cut back on our dinners consequent to the liquid calories we drink with them. Instead, think of liquids' as above and beyond calories. Whenever possible, don't drink your calories. If you worry about vitamins, eat fruit. If you worry about bones and calcium, certainly you can eat dairy, but you can also have almonds, dark leafy greens, tofu, beans, and canned salmon (or you might focus on the likely more important bone health factors of supplemental vitamin D and weight-bearing exercise). Your goal with liquid calories is a simple one—have the smallest number of them you need to like your life but please don't feel that caloric beverages are required healthy living choices, as I'm not aware of a beverage whose health benefits outweigh its calories. ◉

STORAGE

Whether it's preportioning a bulk purchase of nuts into snack packs, using Tupperware to freeze your own versions of frozen dinners, or even investing in a home vacuum sealer to help keep frozen foods at their freshest, organization is a powerful ally, and these simple tools are a great help. Especially if you're just starting out with this, you'll want a wide variety of sizes so that you can try out different storage methods and figure out what works best for your particular lifestyle. It's that whole Boy Scout motto thing about being prepared. Resealable plastic bags, rigid plastic containers, twist-tie bags—get a little bit of everything, because you'll be using them all.

CLOTHING

Despite the fact that exercise doesn't burn enough calories to be a weight loss system all on its own, it's still definitely a part of healthy living. Studies on long-term weight maintenance, including many coming out from the National Weight Control Registry, point to exercise as one of the primary drivers of keeping weight off. I'll get into the science of why later, but for now, think about what comfy clothes you're going to want to wear while you get your body moving. They don't need to be made of Lycra or Spandex, but ensuring you've got clothes on hand in which you'd be comfortable expending some energy is important. Shoes, too. And if you don't have shoes you can walk in, or clothes you can sweat in, it's probably worth a quick trip to the mall. Who doesn't feel better with some new (or newly repurposed) outfits?

CLEAN UP!

This Reset is about giving yourself a fresh start. At the very least, take some time today to make your kitchen sparkle, and if you're ambitious, you might want to consider cleaning and organizing your kitchen cupboards as well. As these first 10 Reset days go by, remember that it's easier to keep things clean than to let things pile up and overwhelm you. Given the fact that it's far easier to lose weight in your kitchen than it is in your gym, ensuring you treat yourself to a clean and welcoming workspace will stack your deck that much further, and the more you cultivate the habit of making your kitchen one of your healthy living sanctuaries, the more you'll want to spend time there. So if you dirty a dish, either wash it immediately or throw it in the dishwasher. Don't let something as easily avoidable as a dirty kitchen interfere with your Reset.

End of Day Checklist

(If you've missed anything, restart Day 1 again tomorrow, and don't spend even a moment beating yourself up about it—life happens. But honestly, if every box isn't ticked, resist the urge to rush ahead and just work on ensuring each and every box is ticked by the end of the day tomorrow.)

- ☐ Your food shopping is done
- ☐ You purchased scales
- ☐ You have storage options ready
- ☐ You have clothing on hand
- ☐ Your kitchen is clean
- ☐ Your journal/app/website is set up
- ☐ You congratulated yourself on being 10 percent Reset

DAY 2: DIARIZE!

So you've got yourself organized and ready to go. Today you're going to start a diary.

Start of Day Checklist
◉ You're prepared to weigh and measure foods and record in real time

I know you've done it before, and it's possible you even hated it, but my experience with thousands and thousands of folks just like you has taught me that whether you end up loving or hating your food diary is all about attitude.

Before we get to food, though, let's talk about money. Have you ever lived with a budget? I know I have. Let me ask you another question. Before you buy stuff, do you look at the price tag? And if you really wanted to maximize your tight budget, and you did plan on looking at price tags, do you think that actually keeping track of your spending in a daily budget ledger would be a good idea? I'm pretty sure you'd agree that the answers to those questions are "Of course!" Because after all, if the budget's tight and you can't afford every single thing you want, keeping careful track of what you buy will protect you from unknowingly overspending.

So should food be any different? For all intents and purposes, from the perspective of weight the currency you have to spend is calories. The higher the calories, the more "expensive" the food will be weight-wise, and consequently if you consider weight to be something that matters to you, looking at foods' price tags is probably a good idea. But just as with money and tight budgets, even if your weight concerns you, and even if you do look at caloric price tags, that doesn't mean you can't buy "expensive" food, food that's higher in calories. It just means you've got to pick and choose those foods and circumstances that make calorically expensive foods worth their calories.

I'm sure you see where I'm going with this: enter the food diary. It's not there to judge you, it's there to guide you and to help you be more conscientious. It's there to provide you with more information about your dietary decisions, because the more information you have before you make any decision in life, the better that decision will be, and the same is certainly true regarding food, calories, and weight. That doesn't mean that you can never decide to consume high-calorie meals or foods, just that you're committed to actually thinking about whether or not they're truly worth it to you.

Careful record keeping can also help you to understand the scale better. More often than not, people believe that weight loss can—and should—be rapid. Keeping a careful food diary and knowing the calories you're consuming can help to take the mystery out of whether the scale ought to be going up, going down, or staying the same.

Folks who believe they ought to be losing much faster might be those very same folks who can't understand why their savings aren't growing faster. If they were to keep careful track of their spending, they would be certain to discover exactly how they're spending more money than they're earning. By keeping a careful budget, they may well be able to shift the balance to savings. It's important to remember, though, there's a limit to how much a person can save, as some expenses simply can't be avoided. Similarly, there's a limit to how much a person can lose, as food plays many real and formative roles in our lives. To put this another way: you can't stop paying your rent or your mortgage any more than you can stop eating dinners.

I don't want you to actually change anything today. If money's tight at home and you can't figure out why, the first step you'd likely take would be to keep a home budget or ledger to sleuth out your current spending patterns. Chances are, there will be at least one area where you're spending far more than you ever would have imagined. But ultimately, you can't figure out what to change until you actually know what you're doing. And so today, while I do want you to keep a food diary, it'll mainly be there just to see what "right now" looks like.

Before we get into how to actually keep your food diary, and how to keep it from driving you crazy, some brief but important food diary background. I want to emphasize that there is perhaps no single behavior that has more value to successful weight management than keeping a careful food diary. Studies on food diarizing make this very clear—folks who keep food diaries lose twice as much weight as those who don't.[1] And those are all-comers studies, meaning that included in those results are folks who weren't particularly wonderful at diarizing. Speaking from my personal experience of having worked with thousands and thousands of folks who have kept food diaries, I'll go further and state that folks who keep their food diaries carefully will lose three times as much weight as folks who aren't diarizing. Working with so many people on food diaries, I'm also well aware that food diaries pose some unique challenges to traumatic dieting's veterans; for many of you, food diaries have horrible associations. Over the years you've likely used food diaries as bludgeons to beat yourselves with; whether over portions, choices, or calories, they've served as your judge and jury.

The thing is, to be useful, food diaries simply can't be used for judgment. They can't be used to tell you if you've been "good" or "bad," or "how much you're allowed," or "how much room is left for dinner." Yet almost invariably, that's how they're adopted.

Ultimately, food diaries are there for guidance, not judgment. Meaning they're not to be used to judge your past decisions. They're there to help to guide your future decisions, because knowing where you're at and where you've been gives you incredibly valuable information that you can utilize in making the decision of whether the food you're considering is actually worth its calories.

Of course, it's not just that food records provide people with information on calories. They have two far more important roles. First, they serve as a great investigational tool. A well-kept food record will provide you with a great deal of information to help understand your dietary choices. More often than not, if you're struggling with hunger or crav-ings, explanatory patterns can be seen in the food record. Once a pattern is identified, it's much easier to correct, and over the course of your Reset, we'll go over some of the most common craving- and hunger-inducing patterns.

To give you an example, let's take my wife's last pregnancy. For some reason, she was much hungrier than with her other pregnancies. Without my suggesting that she do so, she decided to use a food diary to try to suss out what might be going on. Within a week or so, she found the culprit. It was cereal. When she had cereal for breakfast, she was much hungrier later in the day than when she had eggs and toast, despite both break-fasts having roughly the same number of calories and the same quantity of protein (it was a protein-fortified cereal). Once she stopped with the cereal and turned to other sources of breakfast calories and protein, she was right back in control and no longer being pushed around by stomach and brain hungers.

You might notice that on the days you exercise, your hunger and crav-ings are different. Seeing that reflected in a food diary that also tracks cravings or hunger will help alert you to pay more attention to ensuring proper sports nutrition. If you're a shift worker, you may find that on the days you work the late shift, your sugar cravings are stronger. Seeing that on paper may alert you to the need to eat a few hundred calories more on the late days, to help prevent yourself from going overboard with a physi-ologically driven 1,000 craving calories.

The food diary's other most important, and probably most forgotten, role is in habit formation. It takes a great deal of time for a new behavior to be forged into a habit—a behavior that persists effortlessly even in the face of a major life upheaval. Yes, I know there's this belief out there that it takes 21 days to forge a new habit. That belief stems from the work of a plastic surgeon named Maxwell Maltz in his book *Psycho-Cybernetics*, where he described how it took amputees 21 days to stop feeling phan-tom sensations from their missing limbs. Maltz then extrapolated that into the recommendation that a person need spend only 15 minutes a day consciously focusing on their new behavior in order to turn it into a habit. Recent research coming out of University College London from Philippa Lally and her colleagues demonstrated a much more variable response to habit formation; they observed that it took their study's participants between 18 and 254 days to either habitually drink a daily glass of water or do 50 sit-ups before breakfast.[7] My belief is that real habits take years to truly forge, though of course, the more time that passes, the less conscious reinforcement and effort they take to sustain. And that's really what's required in forging a habit: consciously reminding yourself, over and over again, for a very long time, exactly what it is you're trying to remember to do. And every time you write in it, the food diary serves not only to track what you're eating, but those few seconds of writing also serve to remind you of everything else you're trying to do. In so doing, it serves as the behavioral change scaffolding you need to truly build new habits.

Once you get used to keeping a food record, it will likely take a maximum of three to five minutes a day. As I noted earlier, folks who keep food diaries well will, in my experience, lose three times as much weight as folks who don't. So here's three minutes a day that will consciously remind you of your new behaviors and subsequently forge your new habits, and those same three minutes will lead you to double or triple your weight loss. Truly, I can't think of a more valuable behavior or a better weight management friend.

Again, today, I don't want you to make any drastic changes. Instead I think it would be very useful for you to see what life looks like right now. It's likely that there'll be surprises in both directions. Some foods may have far fewer calories than you expect, and some may have far more.

What do I want you to track?

1. What and how much you ate or drank
2. What time you ate it
3. How many calories were in it
4. When, for how long, and how vigorously you exercised
5. When and how dramatic were any episodes of hunger or cravings (whether you succumbed or not); rank these on a scale of 1 to 10

6. Any emotions, thoughts, or concerns that you feel are relatable to food

7. Any triggers you can identify linked to dietary struggle

YOUR DDD SCORE

One of the food diary's most important roles is that of investigator. By looking for trends, you'll be able to troubleshoot more personally what matters to your body, because even though I'll be making recommendations that seem to work for the majority of folks, there's a wide range of normal, and what works for most folks may not work for you.

Integral to you using your diary as a troubleshooter is your DDD or "day's degree of difficulty" score. It's both simple to explain and simple to employ. All you need to do is at the end of each and every day, on a scale of 1 to 10, rank how tough the day was as far as an overall picture that combines hunger, cravings, compulsions, and control. For instance, if you felt rock solid, you made healthy choices all day long, you weren't tempted by indulgences (or if you had indulgences you had only as much as you thought was reasonable), you weren't hungry, and you didn't have any cravings, you might rank your day as a 0, 1, or ?. On the other hand, if you were hungry all day long, had difficulty resisting foods that perhaps in retrospect shouldn't have been worth their calories, if you couldn't possibly "have just one," you might rank your day as a 7, 8, or 9.

By looking back over these rankings and looking for patterns, you'll be able to get a sense of what truly matters to you, which ultimately is how you're going to personalize your approach. While I'll have some very clear-cut and concrete suggestions to start you off, the more detail you put into your food diary, the more useful it will be as an investigational tool that helps you carve out your best lifestyle.

Every scientist knows that the strength of their conclusions depends almost entirely on the robustness of their data collection. Keeping track and subjectively assigning a number to your struggles provides you with crucial information to help determine what works best for you. ☉

WHAT MAKES A FOOD DIARY USEFUL?

Ultimately, two things matter when keeping a food diary: completeness and accuracy, and they're different.

Completeness

You've got to write in foods as you go along. If you wait until the end of the day to try to recall what you've had, studies have shown that you'll forget stuff—portions, choices, or both; maybe not every day, but certainly on some days. Of course, you won't think you forgot anything because, after all, that's what forgetting means. So you have to write the foods down as you eat them. However, you don't need to look up or add up the calories until the very end of the day. Why? Two reasons.

The first reason is time. While it takes only seconds to write down what you've eaten, what does take time is looking up the calories. And if you find the time it takes to look up calories during your busy day is frustrating to you, I'd rather you set the task aside until the very end of the day, rather than flip through a calorie book all day long, get frustrated, quit, and lose the incredibly powerful behavioral change benefit of a six-times-a-day reminder of all of your healthy living strategies.

The second reason is that many traumatic dieting veterans have a difficult time losing the oversimplified and dangerous notion that calories are, in and of themselves, inherently bad. These folks tend to think in terms of calorie ceilings and may well think to themselves, *Crap, I've only got 200 calories left for dinner; I guess I'll have to eat melba toast.* It's about learning from your choices, not blindly limiting them. By looking the calories up at the end of the day, you'll be much less likely to build a false calorie ceiling.

It goes without saying that completeness also means recording the foods that perhaps in previous experiences with food diaries, you simply didn't record because you didn't want yourself or anyone else to see them on paper. If you're not completely honest with your food diary, the only person you're cheating is yourself. It's true, some days your calories are going to be higher than you'd prefer—sometimes for great reasons and sometimes not. But just as life is dynamic, so, too, are your caloric needs. Ultimately, you're aiming for the smallest number of calories you need to be happy each day, and because each day's different, so will your calories be. Some days you're just going to need more calories than others to be happy. I'm guessing the best you can do calorically on my birthday will be much better than the best you can do calorically on yours.

Accuracy

Human eyeballs don't weigh or measure well. You need to use kitchen scales, measuring cups, and measuring spoons. But it's important to note, they're not there to limit you. They're not there to tell you how much you're allowed; they're there to tell you how much you've had. You're the boss, not a cup.

THE DAY I REALIZED I WAS EATING AN EXTRA SNICKERS BAR A DAY

A few years ago, I decided to improve on my own food diarizing accuracy by purchasing an additional digital scale to use at work. Boy, was I surprised. Within a few days, it was saving me a Snickers bar a day in calories! As it turned out, the oranges I had mistakenly believed were "medium-size," in fact weighed nearly double what my calorie book suggested a medium-size orange ought. Consequently, my calories were off by 40 per orange. It also turned out that my small handful of peanuts, when weighed and calculated, contained 100 calories more than an equally small handful of almonds. With some days including two oranges and two handfuls of peanuts, I was regularly missing 280 calories a day from my records—the same number of calories you'll find in a regular-size Snickers bar. More astoundingly, the amount of time it took me to figure that out was on the order of 30 seconds of additional effort in weighing a day, whereas to burn those 280 calories, I'd have had to do an extra 30 *minutes* of hard-core exercise. So not only is this a story about why having a good scale makes such a difference; it's also a cautionary tale about how important it is to track accurately! ◉

Remember, if you underestimate your calories by 20 to 30 percent because you're relying on eyeball measures and recording at the end of the
day, you're not likely to lose much—if any—weight.

BEST PRACTICES

Find a Way to Like It
The people who do the best with food diaries are the ones who enjoy
keeping them. More often than not, these are the folks who refuse to let
the diaries judge them but rather use their diaries to collect information
and inform their decisions. They may even treat it like a game—them
versus calories, or them versus the food industry, where they try to find
ways to keep calories lower without sacrificing the pleasures of food.

Remember, It's the Big Picture That Matters Most
The best diarizers use their diaries to help look for meals they want to
tweak to lower calories, or ones that aren't good enough to be worth their
caloric costs. They tend to focus more on their weekly averages than their
day to day or meal to meal, and they recognize that some days and weeks
are going to be much higher than others.

Be Consistent, Not Perfect
Diary masters tend to keep their records consistently, meal in and meal
out. If they do happen to miss one, they don't simply stop for the rest of
the day, but rather pick up where they left off and do their best to try to
recall the meals they didn't record in real time. Don't fall into the trap
of quitting if your day is incomplete with the plan being *I'll start again
tomorrow*. The people who do that are often the folks who tell me, "I'm
great until lunch or dinner and then it all falls apart." What happens
with them is their perfectionist tendencies have them feel that unless the
day's complete, they're better off waiting until the next day to resume
their record keeping. The problem is that by giving themselves permission to wait until the next day (or worse yet, the next Monday) to resume,
what they're also doing is giving themselves permission to not record,

and every time you give yourself permission to not do something, it'll be that much easier to give yourself that permission again. What those people should be doing the second they recognize that they haven't been recording is start again right then and there. By doing it that way, they'll be reinforcing the habit of recording, rather than reinforcing their own permission not to bother.

Don't Be Shy

If you'd like to be great at food diarizing, but you're shy about keeping one publicly, you've got two options. The first is to ask yourself how you might react if your friend pulled out a food diary after a meal and wrote things down. Chances are, if anything you'd be curious as to what they were doing, and if when you asked they answered that they were keeping track of what they were eating because they were trying to improve their health, I doubt you'd think any less of them—quite likely, you'd be impressed. But if that's not your style, then it may be worth considering an electronic means of recording.

DO 3,500 CALORIES REALLY MAKE OR BREAK A POUND?

The short answer is no. While clinicians have been using the convention of 3,500 calories representing a pound for decades, the fact of the matter is that we are not simply walking math formulae. Experientially, we all know that person who can eat whatever they want and not gain weight, or the person who can seemingly spin around in a circle a few times, clap, and lose. While indeed we can describe food in terms of caloric units of energy, what matters to our bottom lines (and our bottoms) is the energy our bodies are able to utilize from our foods (we can call these *bioavailable calories*), as well as whether or not a food is inherently more or less filling. Unfortunately, there are no tests that can be run to reveal our own internal individual caloric efficiencies, and so despite calories being an imperfect measure, they're the benchmark we'll need to utilize until someone finds a means to measure *bioavailable calories*. ◉

HOW MUCH TIME'S INVOLVED?

At the beginning, I'd mentally budget up to 20 minutes a day, with the bulk of that time spent looking things up. Within a month or two, that should be down to five minutes or less a day. Why? Because the vast majority of us are rather boring eaters, and we eat the same things over and over again with the same meals and snacks rotated over different days. I'd bet most of us don't have more than 40 different meals and snacks in our regular rotations, and if you record them enough times you'll know all of their numbers by heart. Once you get to that point, keeping a food diary will take you two to three minutes a day total. Yet from a weight management perspective, I'd argue that those two to three minutes a day would likely have the same or better weight management benefits as would spending an hour a day in the gym.

Another way to speed things up, especially if you eat the same meals and snacks on a repetitive or ongoing basis, is to use acronyms. A simple capital *B* may suffice for breakfast if you eat the same breakfast every morning. Or if you have two or three breakfasts, you can have B1, B2, and B3. Almonds as a snack might be recorded as "As." So long as you can understand what you've written, you can use any form of shorthand that works for you.

How much time would it take you to write a capital *B*?

For the folks using online services (such as sparkpeople.com, myfit nesspal.com, fitday.com, livestrong.com, and many, many more), while there might be some initial time to set things up and enter your foods for the first time, once they're in your database it may take only as much time to record as it does to pull down a drop-down menu and click a button. Setting your tracker as your computer's home page can also help to remind you to use it. Things are similar with smartphone apps; certainly, the first few days or weeks of entering in your regular food items may be time consuming. But once entered, recording will be as simple as selecting from a pull-down menu or a first-letter search.

Free online calorie databases like the one found at calorieking.com can also be exceedingly helpful in calculations. If you've taken the time to record an accurate measurement, rather than doing your own

FOOD DIARIES ARE EASY TO KEEP
BUT DIFFICULT TO KEEP WELL

Given the incredible access we have to food, the lack of caloric information in many restaurants, the reluctance of most folks to weigh and measure what they're eating, and the nibbles and bites we may randomly have, accurate record keeping can be difficult.

A study done a decade ago helps to illustrate how even trained professionals can stumble with a food diary.[3] Simply designed, the study compared the calories recorded in seven-day food diaries with the calories actually consumed. Half of the subjects were registered dietitians, while half were plain old folk, with the assumption being that the dietitians would be record-keeping ringers.

The results?

First, the nondietitians. Despite actually keeping food records, they missed 18 percent of the calories they consumed. How many calories is that? If we extrapolate their underestimation over an entire year, they'd have missed the recording of over 40 pounds' worth of calories!

Now for the dietitians. While they missed fewer, they still missed 10.5 percent of the calories they consumed. Due to a small sample size, this wasn't deemed statistically significant, but over a year, were that discrepancy maintained, they'd have missed recording 22 pounds' worth of calories.

At my office we sometimes ask patients to do what we call "science experiments," during which for a one- or two-week period they become as anal about record keeping as they possibly can. Weighing and measuring absolutely everything. Recording food within minutes of eating it and ideally not eating out even once. Almost invariably, patients who felt they were fairly accurate with their records before the experiment find anywhere from 200 to 500 calories they didn't even realize were there. ◉

multiplication or division, head over to CalorieKing. Using the search box on their home page, you can enter each food. Then on the ensuing screen there will be a drop-down menu of different measurement options (ounces, grams, cups, tablespoons, etc.) that will allow you to enter your exact measurements without having to bust out your calculator.

"DO I HAVE TO KEEP A FOOD DIARY FOREVER?"

When people ask me that question, I'll always counter with "So what if you did?" When you're good at food diarizing, it's unlikely to take you more than two to three minutes a day to complete. Seems to me that two to three minutes of daily effort is probably worth a lifetime of ease with weight management. I've kept my food diary up for years and honestly, at this point, it's just something I do; I barely think about it.

The truth is, some people will need to keep a diary forever—and there's really no way to guess who that'll be. For whatever reason, some people seem to struggle to keep their caloric intake and choices in check without one. On the other hand, I've also met some folks who after losing their weight through complete and accurate record keeping quit recording and maintained their losses.

Ultimately, though, it's a two- to three-minute intervention that will dramatically improve the likelihood of your long-term success. If weight's something you personally feel is important to keep an eye on, if you can't find two to three minutes a day to put toward yourself, it's probably worth trying to explore the reasons why, as two to three minutes of minor effort shouldn't be overwhelming. ◉

YOUR OWN PERSONAL FOODSCAPE

What's a foodscape? It's the sum total of all of the meals and snacks that rotate throughout your day-to-day life, and by keeping a food diary, you're sure to quickly learn yours.

For most of us, our foodscapes are smaller than we might imagine. ▶

Four or five different breakfasts and snacks, 5 to 10 meals unique to lunch (the rest being leftovers), and 10 to 20 unique dinners. Of course, there'll be some celebratory and indulgent meals here and there, but for most of us, our basics repeat.

The value in knowing your foodscape's calories is that understanding your foodscape will affect the frequency of your choices. If you have two meals you like equally well, but one has double the calories of the other, you'll likely make it less frequently. Or maybe you'll use that knowledge to start tweaking its recipe or looking for an alternative.

The more you know about your choices' calorie contents, the easier it'll be to control your calories.

You'll also find you have meal-out foodscapes and holiday foodscapes. Knowing which meals on the menus of your favorite restaurants are the best choices for you (assuming their nutritional values are available) will help you better navigate eating out. The same goes for holiday meals and snacks. And that's not to say you're supposed to choose the lowest calorie items on the menu or the holiday table, but rather that you should choose the items with the lowest number of calories on the menu or table that you'll actually enjoy—and knowing the numbers will help inform that call.

It's not about perfection; it's about the best choices you can enjoy. Knowing your foodscape by heart provides you with the knowledge you'll need to make your best decisions. ◉

End of Day Checklist
(If anything's missed, restart Day 2 again tomorrow, and don't spend even a moment beating yourself up about it—life happens.)

- ☐ Your home-cooked foods were all weighed and measured
- ☐ Your food was completely diarized, nonjudgmentally, in real time—good, bad, and ugly, without artificial restrictions
- ☐ You read tomorrow's daily plan and you're ready for it
- ☐ You congratulated yourself on being 20 percent Reset

DAY 3: BANISH HUNGER!

So you've got yourself organized and learned how to diarize. Today you're going to eliminate hunger.

Start of Day Checklist
- ◎ You're prepared to weigh and measure foods and record in real time
- ◎ You're prepared to eat on the clock
- ◎ You're prepared to eat even if you're not in the mood

Second only to breathing, eating and drinking are our most important survival skills, and after hundreds of millions of years of evolution, your body is designed to make sure that you do them. To ensure its survival, there are a few things your body keeps track of when it comes to eating. In a practical sense, you can think of your body as having three gauges or sensors: one for time, one for calories, and one for protein. If any one of those sensors detects something wrong, it sets in motion a series of events that ultimately leads to hunger and/or cravings. You can think of it as a burglar alarm system in which if the time, calorie, or protein trip wire goes off, the body sounds the alarm. On the other hand, if you never let your time, calories, or protein needles go too low, you'll preempt those same hungers and cravings—and preventing hunger and cravings is absolutely essential if you're going to be able to decrease your total daily calories without missing those that are gone.

Unlike an alarm system, though, the body's hunger alarms can't be reset. What I mean is that once you've tripped an alarm, you can't simply enter a code to turn it off. For the majority of folks out there, tripping one of the body's alarms doesn't lead to instantaneous hunger or struggles; tripping one of the alarms tends to lead a person to struggle with portions or choices later in the afternoon, evening, and/or nighttime. There's no compensatory behavior that's going to stop your body from trying to influence your choices once this process has been initiated. So if you've skipped breakfast, simply having a larger morning snack or lunch isn't going to cut it if breakfast skipping is one of your personal hunger triggers.

What that means is that organization is far more important to success than sacrifice.

So let's review the three most common integral alarms.

TIME

Your body keeps track of time, and more to the point here, it keeps track of when you've eaten.

For most, the first trip wire is breakfast, and you simply can't wait too long after waking before you eat it. Later than 30 to 60 minutes post waking up, and it's no longer going to be breakfast, it's going to be a morning snack. While I'm not aware of any studies that look at whether a delayed breakfast affects hunger differently than a prompt one, my clinical experience with thousands of patients would suggest that it does—sometimes dramatically. Leave it too long and, paradoxically, your evenings may well become more challenging in terms of cravings and control.

I know, some of you are groaning because you don't feel like eating when you wake up. You're not hungry in the mornings, you might even feel nauseous when you try, and you believe that you just can't keep the food down. Maybe you're the classic breakfast skipper, early morning small snacker, try-to-eat-a-healthy-ish luncher. If you're skipping morning meals, there's no doubt you're a person who consumes the vast majority of their calories late in the day. That pattern of eating will by its very nature lead you to not have the urge or drive to eat when you wake up, as you may well have had a full day's worth of calories from 4:00 p.m. onward the day before.

In the National Weight Control Registry—that research population in which the average registrant has lost 67 pounds and kept them off for five and a half years—78 percent report eating breakfast daily.[1] For registrants, it would certainly seem that breakfast is a cardinal behavior of successful weight management. So if you're keen to finally conquer food, it's likely something you're simply going to have to do.

Remember, the more weight you want to permanently lose, the more of your life you're going to have to permanently change. Eating frequently is a big-ticket change, where big-ticket changes have dramatic consequences.

"DO I REALLY NEED TO EAT SIX TIMES A DAY?"

The simple answer is "no," but simple and practical aren't always the same.

Having worked with thousands of people, I've found the "eat frequently" approach to be the most readily adoptable, as less-frequent meals and snacks require fairly large breakfasts, which seem to be many people's sticking points. However you should know that there are folks out there who are quite comfortable intermittently fasting, eating single daily meals, or splitting things up into three meals a day with no snacking at all.

I think you need to do what's right for you, and using your diary to track cravings, hunger, and calories, you're welcome to experiment on your own. But wait until after these first 10 days. And even if you're reticent to eat so frequently, consider these first 10 days the data set you'll need in order to have a fair comparison with whatever other pattern you'd like to try.

As far as the medical literature goes, there's evidence to suggest that small frequent meals are helpful, and there's also evidence to suggest that they're not. I think in part this contradiction is due to different definitions of snacking and different dietary approaches. It's probably also due to the fact that we're all individuals, and there's a huge degree of variation among us. ⊚

Following breakfast, the rest of the day's pretty straightforward. For the sake of this Reset, I'm going to ask you to not go any longer than three and a half hours without eating; my aim during this Reset period is to put you back in food's driver's seat, where you control it and it doesn't control you. To get there, you need to make sure your hunger and cravings are silenced, and eating frequently, especially including protein and ensuring you have enough calories (we'll get there next, don't worry), will do the trick.

Therefore, to keep this alarm silent you'll have to eat roughly every two and a half to three and a half hours, from the moment you wake up until the moment you go to bed. And yes, if you've got exceptionally long days, you'll require more meals and snacks than those folks who are getting more hours of sleep (but then again, being awake and active also means you're burning more calories).

CALORIES

Your body does track calories. Not as well as you can with a food diary, but it does keep a rough tally.

If you don't have enough calories per meal and snack, again, you're setting yourself up for nighttime struggles as your calorie trip wire gets crossed.

The lesson here is that ensuring you eat enough calories is more important than ensuring you don't eat too many. Eating enough calories per meal and snack is crucial to ensuring physiologically driven hunger and cravings don't push you around.

As far as minimums go, with a plan to eat every two and a half to three and a half hours, I'd recommend a bare minimum of 300 to 350 calories per meal and 100 to 150 calories per snack for women and 400 to 450 per meal and 150 to 200 per snack for men. We'll personalize this even further shortly, but for today, at the very least, I need you to ensure you hit your minimums. That point's so important I'm going to repeat it again: I care about making sure you've eaten enough with every meal and snack, so you've got a lower limit but no traumatic upper limit.

HOW MANY CALORIES DO YOU BURN EACH DAY?

It's a crucial piece of information, and it can either be measured or estimated.

In my offices, we measure metabolism by means of a medical instrument called an "indirect calorimeter." What it does is measure the oxygen a person consumes over a given period of time, converts that into calories, and then extrapolates over a day's time. Having measured thousands of people's metabolisms, I can report that most folks' metabolic rates are pretty darn close to what we'd expect if we simply estimated them, with a few outliers on both ends.

Estimating metabolic rate involves plugging some variables into an equation. Important variables include age, weight, height, sex, and activity levels. If you log onto this book's website at TheDietFix.com, you'll find a metabolism calculator to help you out.

In terms of targets, if you're aiming to lose weight, you'll need to eat fewer calories than you burn, but I don't want you to cut your calories off at the knees. It's a rare woman who can be happily satisfied on fewer than 1,400 calories a day and a rare man who can be happily satisfied on fewer than 2,000 calories. For the sake of this Reset, I'd rather you start off with perhaps a few more calories than you need and work your way down, rather than dive right into low-calorie days. ◉

PROTEIN

You probably already know this, but protein is more filling than either fats or carbohydrates for the same number of calories.

What you may not know is that by including protein in a meal or a snack, you will slow the speed with which your body is able to convert co-consumed carbohydrates into simple sugars and absorb them. This delay helps blunt the body's insulin response and helps to prevent larger and more dramatic blood sugar and insulin fluctuations. What I've regularly seen in my office is also fascinating—missing protein in even one meal or snack may well lead to more struggles at night. Have just cereal for breakfast and you might find that your evening is more difficult to control from a hunger or cravings standpoint.

I want you to include protein in every single meal and snack of your day, which will help to ensure that you're maximally full. Protein's inclusion everywhere will also ensure that you've minimized the chances of your body having to endure rapid or dramatic cycling of your insulin and blood sugar levels; if you don't include protein, the more rapid conversion of carbohydrates to sugars might lead you to a larger and more rapid increase in insulin. That rapid increase in the hormone designed to keep blood sugars lower may then cause your body to overshoot the reduction and lead you to recurrent sugar lows, which many have theorized play a role in the generation of hunger and cravings.

Once the first 10 days are down, if you've been careful to track your days' degrees of difficulty by assigning a daily overall value from 1 to 10 for hunger, cravings, and control, you'll be able to experiment on your own to determine how important protein distribution is to you. My experience has taught me: miss protein in a meal or snack and my body's going to know. Remember, you're embarking on a 10-day Reset during which there's nothing you can't do for just 10 days, so even if you're not fully convinced, I want you to try it anyway.

CARBOHYDRATES

For a number of reasons, carbohydrates—more commonly simply referred to as carbs—deserve some special attention. Perhaps foremost among the reasons is that many post-traumatic dieters view them as an absolute enemy.

There's no denying that low-carb diets "work"—they do in fact lead to weight loss. But weight isn't lost simply because carbohydrates are gone. Research shows that people on low-carb diets aren't as hungry, and as a consequence, weight is lost because people on low-carb diets eat fewer calories.

The issue I tend to have with low-carb approaches isn't that they don't get results. The issue I have with low-carb dieting is that when it comes down to it, a great many people simply aren't willing, regardless of weight loss, to live an extreme low-carb life forever. And if you're not willing to live that way forever, whatever weight you lose on that low-carb approach is going to come back.

If you love the low-carb lifestyle, it's important to know that it doesn't appear to be dangerous. While many medical professionals eschew low-carb diets for fear that avoiding carbohydrates will lead people to consume high levels of saturated fat, which will in turn put people at risk, the medical evidence wouldn't agree. From an evidence-based perspective, right now low-carb (and high-fat) appears just as healthy as, or perhaps even slightly healthier than, more traditional low-fat approaches.

PREEMPTIVE HUNGER-FREE EATING

Really, that's the goal for today. I want you to eat in a manner that prevents hunger. The good news is with a focus on increasing protein, and well-timed meals and snacks, hunger can be prevented with what I call "preemptive eating"—eating *before* you ever let yourself get hungry. Because "wait until you're hungry to eat" is likely the worst piece of dietary advice you've ever received.

Why?

As mentioned earlier, in the same way that you're likely to leave the grocery store with a fuller cart if you've gone in hungry, you're likely to eat more and more indulgently if you sit down to a meal hungry. Hunger most assuredly affects our choices.

And therefore if you're sitting down to a meal hungry, it's as if you're going shopping hungry, only now rather than from grocery store aisles you're shopping from plates, your fridge, your freezer, your cupboards, or worse still, from a menu—shop hungry, choose differently, where differently likely means larger portions and/or more indulgent choices.

As far as I'm concerned, hunger doesn't just come from your stomach; it also comes from your brain. Just as there are a myriad of different physiologic pathways to encourage eating, so, too, are there a myriad of different sensations, emotions, and rationalizations built in to encourage us to seek out food, specifically high-calorie food.

Aside from stomach growling, brain growling hunger consists of things like cravings, compulsions, needs for a "taste" of a certain flavor/tartness/saltiness/sweetness, starting to eat something and having difficulty stopping, and in many cases, even overt losses of dietary control and discretion.

When you're hungry, it's not even remotely difficult to eat a full day's calories (or even more) at a single sitting. The good news is, given the world we live in, hunger is 100 percent preventable. If you go out of your way to plan meals and snacks, you can learn how to keep yours at bay and in so doing stay in control of your portions, your choices, and your calories.

One thing to explicitly point out here: for some people, it feels somewhat unnatural to eat when you're not hungry. I know when it comes time for me to snack, part of me still doesn't really want to. Sometimes I might even feel slightly put off or even ever so slightly nauseated at the thought of eating. If that happens to you, trust me, take the first bite and you'll find that feeling disappears almost instantaneously. Remember, too, that "natural" nowadays isn't. Natural would be your body living in a world with tremendous dietary insecurity, because after all, that was the natural course of things for the last 100 million years or so of our evolution. It's just that we've found ourselves in the very unnatural circumstance of having incredibly calorie-dense foods at our constant beck and call, and the natural consequence of eating when you're hungry in this wholly unnatural environment is to eat far too many calories.

In order to prevent hunger, as noted, there are three simple and straightforward considerations.

Timing: Eat every two and a half to three and a half hours.
Protein: Include protein with every meal and snack.
Calories: Minimums matter, maximums don't. Eat too little at a meal or a snack and you'll pay for it later.

Putting it all together, here's a basic hunger prevention strategy born out of my experiences with thousands of patients. Try it and I bet you'll be surprised at how well it works:

- Determine the number of calories you're aiming for in a day by heading over to TheDietFix.com and plugging your age, weight, height, sex, and activity levels into the calorie needs calculator.

  If you're aiming to maintain your weight, use the maintenance number.

  If you're aiming to lose, start by using the 1-pound weekly loss guidance and resist the urge to start faster.
- Eat *at least* one-fifth of your total daily calories with each meal, and at least 150 calories with *every* snack.
- Have breakfast within 60 minutes of waking up.
- Try to ensure you've had at least 20 grams of protein in each meal and 10 grams in each snack. (There are some suggestions for meals and snacks at the end of this book.)
- For every 45 minutes of sustained moderate or vigorous exercise, ensure you add an additional 150 calories either immediately before or after your workout.
- If you're hungry, it's important that you eat more. You're not going to follow any plan that forces you to fight hunger regularly.

Remember, the quality of your calories will count, too—stack your day with liquid or heavily processed calories and you are more likely to still end up battling hunger.

FOR THOSE DESPERATE TO TRY A THREE MEAL, NO SNACK APPROACH

If you feel it's going to be absolutely impossible for you to snack, here's your hunger prevention recipe. The reason it's not the go-to approach, though, is that it truly requires a great deal of calories and protein per meal, and practically and logistically speaking, that's often a challenge from the perspectives of time and liking it.

- Determine the number of calories you're aiming for in a day by heading over to TheDietFix.com and plugging your age, weight, height, sex, and activity levels into the calorie needs calculator.

   If you're aiming to maintain your weight, use the maintenance number.

   If you're aiming to lose, start by using the 1-pound weekly loss guidance and resist the urge to start faster.

- Eat one-third of your total daily calories with each meal.

- Have breakfast within 60 minutes of waking up.

- Ensure that 25 percent of each meal's calories are coming from protein. While there's a calculator on the website, to crunch your own numbers:

   Take your total daily calories and divide by 48.

   That number is the minimum number of grams of protein you need to have with each meal.

- For every 45 minutes of sustained moderate or vigorous exercise, ensure you add an additional 150 calories either immediately before or after your workout.

- If you're hungry, it's important that you eat more. You're not going to follow any plan that forces you to fight hunger regularly. ◉

"I'M TOO BUSY TO SNACK"

Snacking is probably the preemptive eating behavior that people struggle with the most. More often than not it's because people feel that they are simply too busy to snack. Of course, there's a big difference between being too busy to snack and being too busy to remember to snack. Life has a habit of grabbing hold and not letting go. Hectic workplaces, a bunch of kids running around, an afternoon of gardening planned—it's easy to get lost in what you're doing, especially since I'm suggesting that you should be eating before your body ever reminds you it's hungry.

Thankfully, we live in a world that beeps. I recommend that you employ any one (or more) of the multitude of devices that can beep at you to remind you to snack. For many of you, eating was likely a spontaneous affair, and here I am telling you that I want you to eat on a clock.

As far as alarms go, here are some common options:

At home: Kitchen timers, oven timers, microwave timers, spouses, partners, and children

At the office: Outlook reminders

Out and about: Smartphone or cell phone alarms (to which you can assign a specific ringtone), free online text messaging services such as www.ohdontforget.com, or electronic calendar reminders (Google calendars can be trained to do that).

It's also useful to know how long snacking takes; that will depend on the type of snack. Protein bars or 150 calories of cheese or nuts generally take on the order of 60 to 90 seconds to eat. Fruits, on the other hand, take quite awhile longer; if you're always feeling pressured for time with your snacks, make sure to choose options quicker than fruit. Don't forget, too, that there's virtually no protein in fruit, so if fruit's your snack, ensure you have some protein along with it.

One of the fastest snacks around is premixed protein shakes packaged in drink boxes. While definitely not as filling as food-based snacks, these shakes, available in health food stores, pharmacies, and big-box stores like Costco, are also unobtrusive enough to haul out in meetings or consume while chatting with coworkers, clients, or students at your desk.

Lastly, if you do forget to snack and then you remember just before a mealtime, have the snack then and there. It won't affect satiety the same way, and you may still have a difficult time that afternoon or evening with additional hunger or cravings, but by having the snack you're reinforcing the pattern of behavior that you're trying to cultivate into habit: the pattern that has you snacking between meals in the aim of preempting hunger and remaining in control. By forgoing the snack whose timing is off, all you'll be doing is reinforcing your comfort in missing them in the first place, whereas having them late will reinforce having them overall.

A BRIEF WORD ON MINIMUMS VERSUS MAXIMUMS

I know you're likely used to having limits placed either on how much you're eating or on what you're eating. But here I am telling you that I care more about you eating enough calories per meal and snack! That doesn't mean that you can eat as much as you want, as often as you want, and whatever you want without it affecting your weight. It does mean that I know that if you're actually going to succeed in controlling your calories, you can't be hungry, and ensuring you eat enough per meal and snack is a crucial aspect of hunger prevention. If you're hoping for weight loss, clearly what and how much you eat are going to matter. You're going to need to pick and choose when it's worth it to you to indulge, and part of your decision-making process will involve your weight loss goals. I know you've always imagined that weight loss was willpower. What I'm hoping to prove to you is that willpower is the absence of hunger.

End of Day Checklist

(If you've missed anything, restart Day 3 again tomorrow, and don't spend even a moment beating yourself up about it—life happens.)

- ☐ Your home-cooked foods were all weighed and measured
- ☐ Your food was completely diarized, nonjudgmentally, in real time—good, bad, and ugly, without artificial restrictions
- ☐ Your meals each contained at least one-fifth of your total daily recommended caloric aim and at least 20 grams of protein
- ☐ Your snacks each contained at least 150 calories and at least 10 grams of protein
- ☐ You set up reminders to help yourself remember when to eat
- ☐ You ate an additional 150 calories for every 45 minutes you exercised, either immediately before or after your workout
- ☐ You ate more if you were hungry
- ☐ You read tomorrow's daily plan and you're ready for it
- ☐ You congratulated yourself on being 30 percent Reset

DAY 4: COOK!

So you've got yourself organized, learned how to diarize, and eliminated hunger. Today you're going to start cooking!

Start of Day Checklist
(If you aren't ready with all of these, repeat the prior day's program.)

- You're prepared to weigh and measure foods and record in real time
- You're prepared to eat on the clock
- You're prepared to eat even if you're not in the mood
- You're prepared to cook each and every meal and snack for the remaining week (with the exception of your planned meal out)
- You've packed your lunch and snacks for work today
- You've got a recipe picked out for dinner tonight and have the ingredients at home, ready to go (or you're prepared to go to the supermarket today), along with the ingredients and plans for tomorrow's meals and snacks

There's no better way to ensure you know what's going into your body than for you to make it yourself. We'll get to a meal out in a few days, but right now, I want you to focus on cooking.

One of the primary drivers of overweight and obesity in society is our ever-increasing reliance on meals purchased outside the home. What was once just an occasional personal or family treat has become something many of us will do multiple times per week. Between ever-increasing restaurant portions and the fact that restaurants are far more liberal with calories to begin with, cultivating and nurturing a love affair with your kitchen would be a very wise thing to do.

People sometimes forget that cooking doesn't need to be gourmet. How long does it take to scramble some eggs? To spread peanut butter on whole grain bread? To toss a salad and follow it up by boiling water to cook some whole grain pasta, and then spooning on a reheated meat sauce?

Often the folks who report being too busy to cook are the least organized when it comes to shopping. If you're finding cooking to be a challenge, first and foremost ensure that you've got grocery shopping as a scheduled, recurrent weekly event, as it sure is tough to cook if you don't have the ingredients you'd need to cook with.

Next, ensure that your freezer has some emergency meals. Sure they're not likely to be as healthful as meals you've transformed from raw ingredients, but boxed meals are almost certainly better calorically than takeout. Spend some time in the supermarket reading the boxes of different frozen meals, and buy a bunch of the ones that seem appropriate for you calorically and nutritionally. That way, over time you can find three or four you enjoy enough to keep on hand for those inevitable times when you've come in late and the last thing you want to do is cook.

You might also want to consider time-saving devices like a slow cooker that you can load before you leave in the morning, so that when you get home there's something ready and waiting.

Lastly, when you do cook, cook lots. Double or triple all of your recipes. Doing so won't take double or triple the effort, and you'll create your own stock of homemade frozen meals if you immediately pack away the extra into meal-size, labeled portions.

This week, try to find at least one new recipe to try. Getting stuck in a rut of eating "safe" meals, meals whose calories you know and that are easy to control, might be helpful in the short run but isn't likely a strategy you'll stick with for good. That strategy is the classic "meal plan" diet, in which you or someone else comes up with very specific calorie-controlled meals and snacks. Regardless of their safety or even your initial enjoyment of them, if you're stuck without the flexibility to eat a varied diet, you might well quit the approach altogether.

I recommend making one night a week "new-recipe night," as doing so is a great way to encourage variety, improve cooking skill, and avoid monotony. Recruiting your family to help can also encourage family unity and may allow you to teach your children about nutrition without making it about *them*. Find a cookbook that appeals to all of your family members, ideally a cookbook that includes nutritional breakdowns of its recipes, and then each family member can take turns picking that week's recipe.

LUNCHES AND SNACKS

The calories and money you'll save by ensuring you've packed your meals and snacks are so dramatic that they deserve special mention.

The 5 or at the very most 10 minutes that it'll take you to make and pack your lunch and snacks for the next day will have a far greater impact on your long-term weight management success than finding the time to hit the gym. The end of this book provides recipes for breakfast, lunch, and dinner and suggested snacks. The recipes aren't complicated or fancy, and don't require exotic ingredients; they're just good, not-too-time-consuming food that I hope you'll find as delicious as anything you can get from a take-out menu.

COOKBOOKS AND RESOURCES

Thanks to the Internet, there are a great many resources out there. If you do utilize online recipes, make sure to use only ones that provide you with nutritional information—it's a lot easier to keep track of calories if someone's already done it for you!

Cookbook-wise, if you don't already own some with calorie counts and nutritional breakdowns built in, why not spend half an hour leafing through your options at your local bookstore? Find one or two that have all of the information you need, and also have simple-to-follow recipes that appeal to your particular tastes. ◉

It might go without saying, but I'll say it anyway: it's almost certainly easier to pack your lunch the night before than to try to whip things together during a busy morning. My own lunches tend to be a repurposing of the previous night's dinner (we cook large amounts to freeze as well as to pack the next day for lunch), a frozen portion of a dinner meal, or a sandwich along with fruit and/or a salad.

That said, it might also be worth having a basic, if not necessarily incredibly delicious, go-to lunch for when you've forgotten or not bothered and you're flying out the door. My go-to is exceedingly simple: two slices of whole grain bread, an ounce and a half of Havarti cheese, some fruit, and if we have one hanging around, a tomato. I don't bother building the sandwich at home but do so at work, where we also have some mustard in our fridge that I sometimes like to add.

My other lunch rule? I eat lunch out at work only if someone else is buying.

YOU VERSUS THEM

When it comes to meals prepared for you, rather than *by* you, chances are they're going to be prepared in such a way as to make them both irresistible and hyperpalatable. Pulitzer Prize–winning author and *New York Times* investigative journalist Michael Moss, in his book *Salt, Sugar, Fat,* carefully details how the food industry, in a bid to maximize profits, has made a science out of making foods hyperpalatable. His premise, and it's one we've all experienced ourselves, is that the "I bet you can't eat just one" phenomenon is powerfully manipulated by food engineers who carefully tweak amounts of fats, sugars, and salts to make food less resistible. Of course, if it's more difficult to resist, you'll eat more of it, and if you eat more of it, you'll buy more of it. ◉

CALCULATING RECIPE CALORIES

The most basic way to calculate the calories in a given recipe is to total it ingredient by ingredient, then figure out how many servings you've made by portioning out the whole dish and dividing your total number of calories by the total number of servings.

While that's certainly tedious, if you're like me, you won't have that many recipes to calculate. So long as you stick to the same recipe and portion size every time around, you won't need to recalculate whenever you have that meal. But make sure there's somewhere logical for you to keep track of your calculations. Whether it's in your cookbooks directly or in a folder, notebook, or spreadsheet, just make sure you've got something on hand in the kitchen where you can record your numbers.

If you're calculating manually, let me steer you again to the free resource at www.calorieking.com. With it, you can enter each item one by one, scale them up or down on a variety of different measurement scales by means of a drop-down menu, and then just jot down the numbers for each ingredient. Once you've calculated all the ingredients, add them up and there's your total for the dish. The only thing left for you to do is divide by the number of servings.

Alternatively, you can get a number of calories for the entire dish, then use your kitchen scale to weigh out the portions and use that number to calculate calories by portion weight. While this may be a touch more difficult mathematically, if you can calculate the calories per ounce, it'll allow for greater accuracy in tracking. As always, I'll point out: the scale isn't there to tell you how much you're allowed, but rather there to help you to record how much you decided to have.

A higher tech way would be to use an online service or a computer program. A quick Google search for "recipe calorie calculator" will bring up a pile of options. You should try a few out before deciding which you like best. What those programs will do is both serve as recipe databases, and allow you to tweak and modify recipes to determine the impact on calories of different ingredient substitutions or portion changes. For example, we use Mastercook at home. I remember once plugging in a ▶

summer burger recipe that had been a semiregular staple—and I was flabbergasted to learn the calories per burger. Once I knew how many there were, I decided to shrink the size of the burgers, making six rather than four. Doing this got the calories down to a number that seemed more reasonable, and I wasn't any hungrier! Had I not been able to knock the number down, or if even at six servings it were ridiculously high, I'd probably have dropped it from our rotation altogether because while the burgers are good, they're not *that* good.

An easy way to calculate your recipes may be to crunch two recipes a day on the weekend and keep a spreadsheet, or write the numbers directly into your cookbooks. Figure it'll take you at most three minutes a recipe, and chances are within two to three months, you'll have the bulk of your dinners done. Chances are, too, that there will be surprises in both directions—meals that are surprisingly low or high in calories, which in turn may affect how often you choose to make them and the size of your preferred portions. ◉

YOU, COOKING

Aside from beverages, for the rest of your Reset period (excepting your planned night out), I want you to ensure that nothing passes your lips that you didn't either make from scratch yourself or purchase in the supermarket (not, though, from the restaurant-style take-out section that many supermarkets now have).

Take 20 to 30 minutes today to map out your meals for the rest of your Reset. Then create a shopping list for the ingredients you need. Determine and schedule when it would fit for you to go and pick up your items. To make your life easier, I recommend that unless you plan on going the dinner leftover route for your lunches, tonight you should also assemble the rest of your week's lunches, and plan out and preportion your workweek's snacks (for instance, if you're going to snack on almonds, prepack some small plastic bags with the portion of your choosing).

Again, remember, it need not be gourmet! If you're not particularly comfortable in the kitchen, give yourself time to learn and to grow, and start with what you know. If you're stuck for ideas, head to the back of the book for some easy favorites of mine.

MIXING, POURING, ADDING, AND STIRRING AIN'T COOKING

As far as health goes, it may be the food industry's most destructive legacy: this notion that "home cooking" can consist of mixing packets, jars, and boxes together.

It's an incredibly pervasive notion, too.

Some examples:

- Take box of dehydrated frozen refined flour noodles. Boil water. Add contents of box. "Cook." Open jar of sauce. Add sauce.

- Brown meat of choice. Add packet of "flavoring." Stir. Serve over store-bought buns, wraps, or rehydrated noodles.

- Take box of frozen "food" of choice. Microwave or heat in oven. Optional: serve alongside baked bagged french fries.

- Take ready-made pizza out of box. Heat in oven.

- Mix package of brown powder with eggs and water. Put in cake pan. "Bake."

I could go on.

When I meet new patients, I'll always go through their eating-out history, but rarely their *eating-out-eating-in* history, and I probably should.

Those examples up above? They'll get me as close to actual cooking as watching movies will get me to winning an Oscar.

Cooking, *actual cooking,* is the transformation of raw ingredients. And there's definitely something special about actual cooking. A sense of accomplishment, of healthfulness, of basic goodness—even when cooking nutritionally less than stellar meals.

Sadly, over the years, the food industry has aimed to co-opt that something special, literally designing foods that require only the most ▶

basic of input and effort so as to perpetuate the gigantic white lie that we're "home cooking."

Is there a meal in your home you've unfairly labeled "home-cooked"? If there is, how about trying to actually cook it at home this week? It may well be easier than you think, and guaranteed, it'll be far more rewarding. ◉

End of Day Checklist

(If you've missed anything, restart Day 4 again tomorrow, and don't spend even a moment beating yourself up about it—life happens.)

- ☐ Your home-cooked foods were all weighed and measured
- ☐ Your food was completely diarized, nonjudgmentally, in real time—good, bad, and ugly, without artificial restrictions
- ☐ Your meals each contained at least one-fifth of your total daily recommended caloric aim and at least 20 grams of protein
- ☐ Your snacks each contained at least 150 calories and at least 10 grams of protein
- ☐ You set up reminders to help yourself remember when to eat
- ☐ You ate an additional 150 calories for every 45 minutes you exercised, either immediately before or after your workout
- ☐ You ate more if you were hungry
- ☐ You cooked all of your meals and snacks today
- ☐ You mapped out the rest of your Reset meals and have both created a shopping list and added your trip to the supermarket to your schedule
- ☐ You read tomorrow's daily plan and you're ready for it
- ☐ You congratulated yourself on being 40 percent Reset

DAY 5: THINK!

S o you've got yourself organized, learned how to diarize, eliminated hunger, and started to cook. Today you're going to learn how to ask the world's two most important questions, and in so doing, learn to think differently!

Start of Day Checklist
(If you aren't ready with all of these, repeat the prior day's program.)

- You're prepared to weigh and measure foods and record in real time
- You're prepared to eat on the clock
- You're prepared to eat even if you're not in the mood
- You're prepared to cook each and every meal and snack for the remaining week (with the exception of your planned meal out)
- You've packed your lunch and snacks for work today
- You've got a recipe picked out for dinner and have the ingredients at home, ready to go (or you're prepared to go to the supermarket today), along with the ingredients and plans for tomorrow's meals and snacks
- You're prepared to put some time aside and think about exactly what it is you're trying to accomplish, and why

SETTING UP YOUR NEW IDENTITY

By now you've made some real changes!

You're nonjudgmentally keeping track of what you're eating. You're preparing your own meals and snacks. You're eating to provide yourself with physiologic freedom from hunger. And you're keeping yourself stocked with everything you need to continue these new behaviors.

These may seem like small steps, but after decades of walking on unsteady ground, small steps are a great plan. Really, what these small steps are walking you towards is a new identity—a new healthy identity that you can take true pride in, and a life free from traumatic dieting.

Today's all about figuring out just who exactly the new you is. It's not a trivial exercise, as holding onto beliefs about yourself that are self-destructive may lead you to sabotage your own best efforts. You've gotten to this point in the book because you've realized that things need to change, and the behaviors and identities that got you here are no doubt part and parcel of what's been holding you back and what's got to go. What we need to do together is work on forging you a new identity, one that you can rightfully take pride in, and one that banishes traumatic dieting forever.

The reason how you identify yourself is so important is because identity is a powerful creature. If you identify yourself a certain way, straying from that self-perceived belief system will be uncomfortable. For instance, if you identify yourself as "an honest person," lying will make you very uncomfortable. But what if you identify yourself as someone who "doesn't live a healthy life" or as a "perfectionist," or as someone who's highly self-critical? I don't want you to challenge yourself with a self-fulfilling negative prophesy; I want you to become a self-fulfilling positive one—one that doesn't care what you weigh. Because regardless of your actual weight, you can indeed live a healthy life if you respect and admire the fact that you're doing your personal best. It doesn't matter if you have more weight than a body mass index table or an ideal weight chart tells you you should. Weight does not preclude living a healthy lifestyle. Living a healthy lifestyle involves making the healthiest dietary choices you can enjoy. After all, the nonsmoker who's only five days past their last puff may not be on as steady a footing as they'll be five years on, but they're still a nonsmoker!

Your footing's bound to get more certain. But for now, it's worth taking a moment of pride for embarking on this new journey, one that's definitely not going to be "perfect."

Is there any area of your life other than your weight where your personal best wouldn't be good enough? Yet for years you've likely berated yourself for not losing faster, not losing more, not exercising more, not being stricter, not suffering enough. Well, that stops today. From this day forward you're going to identify yourself as a person grounded in reality, and reality allows for imperfection. To strive to be ideal at anything immediately sets you up for failure.

So what does "personal best" mean?

If we're talking about weight and food, it means eating the smallest number of calories you need to honestly enjoy your day. Without a doubt, some days will require more calories than others to be enjoyed! The only limits to your daily calories are the lower limits representing bare minimum numbers of calories you must eat in each meal and snack. There are no maximums, and some days are going to be high. Sometimes those days will come with good reasons (holidays, vacations, birthdays, etc.), and sometimes they'll come with preventable reasons (missed meals or snacks, lack of protein). Remember that even on those days when you might have hunger and might crave higher calories or more indulgent choices, or when more indulgent choices are wholly appropriate to the day, you can still do your best. Sure, your best might involve some very high-calorie and not remarkably healthful choices, but there will still be a best choice to be made. It's just that the options from which you're choosing on a hungry or a celebratory day may not be as healthful as the options you'd have considered if you weren't hungry or it weren't a celebration.

Exercise-wise, it also means exercising only as much as you can honestly enjoy. Some days you won't be able to enjoy any, and some days, only very small amounts.

Weight-wise, it means that rather than talking about your ideal weight, or some body mass index, or your body fat percentage, instead you're talking about your "best" weight, where your best weight is whatever weight you reach when you're living the healthiest life that you can honestly and realistically enjoy. Even if you've still got weight to lose, even if the scale is still reading a higher number than you'd like, knowing you're doing the best you can to manage it is phenomenal, laudable, and worthy of self-congratulatory praise.

I don't expect this aspect of your new identity to come easily, but I'm guessing that if you're this far Reset, you're rationally ready to tackle this next step.

If you've spent years traumatically dieting, you might be worried about how long you'll be able to make this plan work. If you're discouraged by the fact that your weight's not where you want it, or if you're having difficulty taking pride in your first small steps, pretend that you're counseling your closest friend or relative who's just taken those very same small steps to try to improve their attitudes and lifestyles. Whatever you would tell them, I want you to tell yourself, because learning to treat yourself with as much love and respect as you treat your friends and family is crucial. Why wouldn't you deserve those same considerations?

THE WORLD'S TWO MOST IMPORTANT QUESTIONS!

Have you ever thought about the fact that our brains tend to interpret our lives through internal questioning? Whatever's going on in our lives, to help understand it our inner monologues start off with inner questions.

Unfortunately for many, our internal inquisitors are both monotonous and merciless, asking the same few questions over and over again. Questions like:

What's wrong with me?
Why can't I just do this?
What's my problem?

The brain, well, it's a very accommodating organ. If you ask your brain a question, it'll deliver an answer. And if the question by its very nature asks you to find fault with yourself, you can bet your bottom dollar that your brain will deliver—usually in the form of an emotional beat-down the likes of which you would never deliver to any other human being. And those questions, they're all questions asking for negative answers. More to the point here, they're the very same questions that we tend to ask ourselves following any slip off our wagons or bumps in our roads.

It doesn't really matter which wagon or road it is. Whether we're working on our weight, our relationships, or our jobs, life isn't a straight line and neither are our efforts. Some weeks, frankly, we all occasionally blow things without any good reason.

Has shaming and blaming yourself for failure ever helped motivate you to ultimately succeed? I doubt it; my guess is that those recurrent negative thoughts are what have led you in the past to eventually stop trying.

Well, from now on, I want you to envision every slip, bump, and challenge as an opportunity. I'm going to ask you to use your more difficult and challenging times, and your natural inclinations to ask yourself questions whose answers by definition are negative, as huge, bright spotlights to illuminate the opportunity to turn things around.

Every time you hear your inner voice start down the self-hate rabbit hole or get into the shaming-and-blaming world, I want you to use that recognition and awareness to simply ask yourself two new questions.

What can I do right now that I can be proud of?
What can I do right now that will help a little bit?

You can apply these new questions to anything, and wielding them is dead simple. If you're unhappy with yourself and the circumstances you find yourself in, or with the way you're reacting to a particular situation, take a step back to think about how you can answer these questions.

If you're working on improving your eating and you're frustrated with what you think was an unnecessary overindulgence, maybe the answers to those questions will be to choose to make a home-cooked, calorie-controlled dinner, or write in a food diary, or go shopping for healthier staples, or pack your lunch for tomorrow, or even take a non–food related but pride-inducing 20-minute walk.

If you're working on improving your relationship and you're in the middle of a fight, pull out the questions; maybe you'll call someone up and tell them you love them, buy somebody some flowers, or make the apology you've been procrastinating over.

Heck, even if you're just stuck in traffic, and you're finding yourself getting unnecessarily and destructively furious about it, maybe the answers are as simple as finding a great song on the radio or taking a moment to reflect on all of those things you're thankful for in life. Life's just too short to let traffic get the best of you.

Bottom line: the situation has stayed the same, but the way you're asking your brain to interpret it has changed. One set of questions is destructive and rear thinking. The other, constructive and forward thinking. It's difficult to build momentum off of negativity, but pride? Pride's powerful.

Pride's so powerful that some people find it helpful to create a pride journal, a place where they keep track of their small victories. Doing so lets them pull it out during more difficult times and quickly see how far they've come.

So those questions again:

What can I do right now that I can be proud of?
What can I do right now that will help a little bit?

Take a moment, too, to be proud of the new identity you're adopting. If everything you thought you knew about weight management and healthy living were true, you wouldn't have been driven to pick up this book. You're breaking free of society's traumatic dieting shackles, and that's something worthy of a good pat on the back. So think about what you're doing, and if there's anything that isn't yet going as well as you think it could, ask yourself your new questions and follow through immediately with your constructive answers.

End of Day Checklist

(If you've missed anything, restart Day 5 again tomorrow, and don't spend even a moment beating yourself up about it—life happens.)

- ☐ Your home-cooked foods were all weighed and measured
- ☐ Your food was completely diarized, nonjudgmentally, in real time—good, bad, and ugly, without artificial restrictions
- ☐ Your meals each contained at least one-fifth of your total daily recommended caloric aim and at least 20 grams of protein
- ☐ Your snacks each contained at least 150 calories and at least 10 grams of protein
- ☐ You set up reminders to help yourself remember when to eat
- ☐ You ate an additional 150 calories for every 45 minutes you exercised, either immediately before or after your workout
- ☐ You ate more if you were hungry
- ☐ You cooked all of your meals and snacks today
- ☐ You asked constructive, not destructive, questions if things weren't going according to plan
- ☐ You recognized that your personal best is great
- ☐ You read tomorrow's daily plan and you're ready for it
- ☐ You congratulated yourself on being 50 percent Reset

DAY 6: EXERCISE!

So you've got yourself organized, learned how to diarize, eliminated hunger, started to cook, and learned how to think differently. Today you're going to learn an eight-word exercise manifesto upon which to build your life.

Start of Day Checklist
(If you aren't ready with all of these, repeat the prior day's program.)

- You're prepared to weigh and measure foods and record in real time
- You're prepared to eat on the clock
- You're prepared to eat even if you're not in the mood
- You're prepared to cook each and every meal and snack for the remaining week (with the exception of your planned meal out)
- You've packed your lunch and snacks for work today
- You've got a recipe picked out for dinner and have the ingredients at home, ready to go (or you're prepared to go to the supermarket today), along with the ingredients and plans for tomorrow's meals and snacks
- You're prepared with constructive questions to deal with potentially destructive circumstances
- You've got exercise shoes and comfortable clothes at the ready

Studies on exercise and weight control are quite clear cut. Folks who exercise are far more likely to keep their weight off than those who don't. Of course, they're also clear on another point. Exercise alone isn't likely to take off much, if any, weight.

A great many traumatic dieters believe heavy-duty or lengthy exercise

is a linchpin for their success; that exercise—high intensity, extended duration, or both—is crucial and that without it, they're finished.

The truth?

Exercise is crucial in weight management, but it's far more important
a factor in keeping the weight off than it is in losing it.

That said, looking at the thousands of people who've completed my office's weight management program, a program that indeed includes exercise, it's not just the folks who are keeping it off that benefit from exercise;
the folks who are exercising the most are usually also the folks who are
losing the most weight.

But didn't I just tell you exercise isn't likely to take off much, if any,
weight? The unfair truth is that exercise doesn't burn nearly as many
calories as would seem fair. To put this in some perspective, you could
lose about a pound running a marathon in three and a half hours or by
walking it in 10 hours. Either way, moving your body consistently for the
26.2 mile distance, you're likely to have burned somewhere in the neighborhood of a pound's 3,500 calories.

How many marathons do you want to run in a week?

I know, I know, I told you that my patients who exercise more lose
more. So if it's not burning enough calories to help you shed those pounds,
what difference is exercise actually making? In my opinion, the biggest
change that exercise brings to your life is to your attitude. Where I see
exercise's role in weight management isn't in the direct calories burned,
though they do provide a bit of a buffer for inaccurately counted or hid-
den calories. In truth, exercise's most important role in weight management is in cultivating a positive attitude towards healthier living. Studies
have demonstrated that those folks in a weight management effort who
are exercising the most tend to consume fewer calories and score higher
on a healthy eating inventory score sheet.[1] Exercise may also help by improving your mood, your sleep, and your stress levels, which in turn will
certainly have a positive impact on your appetite, your drive, and your
energy and may also lower your need to use food to self-medicate.

From a purely caloric perspective, and ignoring the psychological
benefits of exercise, figure the dietary component of your lifestyle is re-

sponsible for 70 to 80 percent of your weight, while your fitness accounts for the remaining 20 to 30 percent. If you're exceedingly active, you may be able to shift those percentages more towards exercise, but most of us don't have the time, energy, inclination, or stamina to sustain that degree of exercise.

So how much exercise should you do?

MY EIGHT-WORD FITNESS MANIFESTO

"Some is good. More is better. Everything counts."

From a medical perspective, there is perhaps no other modifiable determinant of health that has a greater impact on your health than exercise. Being fit and eating a healthful diet, regardless of your weight, is an important goal, with exercise and healthy eating virtually erasing a large percentage of the statistical risks of the weight itself. What that means is that yes, absolutely, a person can be both fit and fat.

The great news about exercise?

Small bits add up.

Unless you're training for an endurance sport, when it comes to weight management, exercise's benefits are cumulative and need not be consecutive.

Think of it like going to the bank. Whether you go once a day and deposit $30, or go three times a day to deposit $10, at the end of the day you're going to have the same amount of money in your account.

One study compared total duration of exercise, improvements in cardiovascular fitness, and weight loss in women who were instructed to go to the gym for 40 minutes three times a week and women who were instructed to take every 10-minute block they could find to do a short bout of exercise.[2]

The results?

The short-bout women actually did more exercise, improved their cardiovascular fitness more, and lost more weight than the long-duration women.

WHAT'S THE BEST TYPE OF EXERCISE FOR WEIGHT MANAGEMENT?

There's no right answer to that question. Ultimately, the best exercise for your weight management effort is the exercise you actually enjoy enough to keep doing.

It can be traditional weight management–style exercising like hitting the gym, jogging, or power walking, but it can also be the nontraditional stuff. I call that "functional exercise," and it's made up of activities you might need to do anyhow. Here are some examples:

- Yardwork. Gardening and snow removal can both be fabulous forms of exercise. Chopping wood, weeding, and deck building certainly aren't too shabby, either.
- Walking the dog.
- Housework. Sweep instead of vacuum, wash dishes by hand, take the clothes out to a clothesline to dry. Home improvement projects like refinishing a table or a chair (if done with manual tools), painting, laying carpet, and drywalling all get the heart going.
- Commuting. If you can bike or walk to work, the store, or your children's school, you'll be far ahead of the game.
- Walk and talk. Whether it's at work in the form of a walk and talk–style meeting, or at home taking a different family member with you on a short evening walk for some quality time, walking's a great time for a chat.

And then there's the other nongym stuff:

- Dancing
- Yoga
- Martial arts
- Weekend bike rides

- Hiking
- Community and fund-raising race events

SO WHAT ARE YOU GOING TO DO TODAY?

Something.

It doesn't matter what you choose to do, so long as mentally you've set aside a specific amount of time to spend on a specific activity with the primary aim of the activity being intentional exercise.

As far as how much you ought to do today? As much as you can enjoy—and in these early days, that may not be a huge amount. What's important isn't the duration of the exercise, it's the intentionality of it.

Whether it's a five-minute walk outside, a few minutes of weeding, dusting off your treadmill, or time spent intentionally engaging in physical play with your children or grandchildren, what's important is that you mentally acknowledge the importance of exercise to your health and at the same time, the importance of not biting off more than you can chew.

Your goal is as much exercise as you can enjoy each day, and while I'm sure virtually every day you can enjoy at least a little bit, some days the most you can enjoy won't be very much at all.

Truly, there is an amount that you can probably do each day without a struggle. I call that amount your "toothbrush level" of exercise; if you've got it in your head that unless you do *x* minutes per day of exercise, it's not worth doing, that'd be akin to thinking that unless you brush your teeth 30 minutes at a shot it's not worth brushing.

My eight-word manifesto for exercise is pretty straightforward, and given all the data piling up on the risks of sitting and the benefits of small bouts of exercise, I'm willing to go out on a limb and suggest it's probably even supported by evidence.

Some is good. More is better. Everything counts.

Your "toothbrush level"? Well, you know exercise has tremendous health benefits. So what amount of exercise do you think you'd be able to add to your day, regardless of likability? Five minutes? Ten?

And then, as with brushing your teeth, figure out when you're going to do it.

Maybe it'll simply be parking five minutes away from work so that you get five minutes of walking on either end of your workday. Maybe it'll be a brief 10-minute weights or calisthenics program when you wake up. Whatever you decide, figure out when you're going to do it, because simply aiming at a nebulous "more" isn't likely to help.

Next, set up a reminder system. Smartphones, Outlook reminders, even old-school hard-copy paper calendars—use them, because here you'll be trying to remember to do something you're not accustomed to doing, and reminders count. How many times do you think your parents reminded you to brush your teeth before you simply started brushing automatically?

I know more is better, but truly, everything counts. Who knows, as your fitness improves and you grow accustomed to intentional daily exercise, perhaps your toothbrush level will grow, too.

Also, don't forget to add your exercise into your food diary. Not calories burned, though. Instead, keep track of the time of day you exercised, its duration, its intensity, and any positive emotions you can hang your hat on, because writing it down is just one more in a series of reminders that you're consciously trying to change your life.

End of Day Checklist

(If you've missed anything, restart Day 6 again tomorrow, and don't spend even a moment beating yourself up about it—life happens).

- ☐ Your home-cooked foods were all weighed and measured
- ☐ Your food was completely diarized, nonjudgmentally, in real time—good, bad, and ugly, without artificial restrictions
- ☐ Your meals each contained at least one-fifth of your total daily recommended caloric aim and at least 20 grams of protein
- ☐ Your snacks each contained at least 150 calories and at least 10 grams of protein
- ☐ You set up reminders to help yourself remember when to eat
- ☐ You ate an additional 150 calories for every 45 minutes you exercised vigorously, either immediately before or after your workout
- ☐ You ate more if you were hungry

☐ You performed at least your toothbrush level of exercise

☐ You cooked all of your meals and snacks today

☐ You asked constructive, not destructive, questions if things weren't going according to plan

☐ You recognized that your personal best is great

☐ You read tomorrow's daily plan and you're ready for it

☐ You congratulated yourself on being 60 percent Reset

DAY 7: INDULGE!

S o you've got yourself organized, learned how to diarize, eliminated hunger, started to cook, learned how to think differently,
and added in some exercise. Today you're going to learn how to
include chocolate.

Start of Day Checklist
(If you aren't ready with all of these, repeat the prior day's program.)

- You're prepared to weigh and measure foods and record in real time
- You're prepared to eat on the clock
- You're prepared to eat even if you're not in the mood
- You're prepared to cook each and every meal and snack for the remaining week (with the exception of your planned meal out)
- You've packed your lunch and snacks for work today
- You've got a recipe picked out for dinner and have the ingredients at home, ready to go (or you're prepared to go to the supermarket today), along with the ingredients and plans for tomorrow's meals and snacks
- You're prepared with constructive questions to deal with potentially destructive circumstances
- You've got exercise shoes and comfortable clothes at the ready, and you have at least your toothbrush level of exercise planned
- You're prepared to eat a food that your prior dieting efforts would have forbidden expressly, and you're prepared to eat it guilt free!

REAL LIFE INCLUDES CHOCOLATE

Real life may include chocolate, but I've met plenty of traumatic dieters who believe that in order to succeed, their lives can't. And chocolate's a tough pill not to swallow, or maybe for you it'd be avoiding ice cream, potato chips, french fries, or pizza. That's probably why I'm willing to wager that I've written more actual prescriptions for chocolate, ice cream, Chinese food, pizza, fried chicken, and potato chips than any other doctor on the planet.

It's tough to out-will hundreds of millions of years of evolution that tells your body it has to stock up on foods high in sugars and fats. Even if you try, eventually your body will win; good luck convincing your body that it should be happy with carrot sticks when it's craving cookies, chips, or ice cream.

While of course there's no such thing as the eat-whatever-you-want, whenever-you-want, as-much-as-you-want weight management plan, blindly cutting out the unhealthy (but often yummy) foods simply isn't sustainable.

PRIMARY AND SECONDARY BINGE EATING

Binge eating is exceedingly common. Studies routinely demonstrate that 30 percent of people seeking help with their weight struggle with binge eating, and as discussed earlier in the book, it can truly be psychologically devastating.

I believe there are two sorts of binge eaters, primary and secondary. If you're someone who struggles with binge eating, there's one question that can often determine by itself which type you are: "Do your struggles have a time of day attached to them?" What I'm asking is whether your struggles tend to occur at or after a particular time of day. If the answer's yes, then I'd bet you're a secondary binge eater. If the answer is, "No, I can binge pretty much any time of day," then you're more likely to be a primary binger.

The difference between primary and secondary binge eating isn't ▶

the amounts eaten or the distress felt. The difference is that secondary binge eating responds dramatically to better dietary organization. With regular meals and snacks ensuring enough calories and enough protein, suddenly, almost magically, the drive to binge disappears, or at the very least markedly dissipates.

Primary binge eaters also tend to respond well to better dietary organization, though there are some who still struggle. These binge eaters may benefit from seeing a psychologist with a special interest in binge eating and might also benefit from the use of medications.

Regardless of whether you're a primary or secondary binge eater, ensuring that you eat enough calories is incredibly important, as restriction is one of the most common binge eating triggers. In my office I usually recommend that binge eaters start at a lower limit of 1,600 calories per day and absolutely must have at least 400 of those calories as part of a protein-rich breakfast. ◉

Ultimately, dieting can't be about denying yourself the foods you enjoy. While that may work for a while, it's certainly not going to work for good. When you finally do allow yourself to have that forbidden food (and you know as well as I do that eventually there'll be a circumstance in which you will), a cascade of traumatic dieting events is likely to unfold.

Tell me if this sounds familiar: Initially there will be that heavenly first bite or two. The one that makes your body scream, *This is sooo good.* This will likely be followed by rapid consumption. You don't know when you'll let yourself eat it again, and it's been so long that the drive to eat is irresistible. Next will come a binge of sorts. The size of the binge will vary, but one thing's for certain: you're not going to be thinking about how much you're eating. The binge may grow and spill over into other forbidden foods as oftentimes the inclusion of one forbidden food will lead you to add another because clearly the day's a write-off, and you figure that since you've already blown it on one forbidden food, you might as well have a few others.

When you're done eating, then an artificially apocalyptic reality is likely to sink in. You're going to feel demoralized and defeated. Guilt and self-loathing will wash over you. You may lash out at yourself, with that awful voice in your head telling you you're a loser. That you've blown it. That you can't succeed and that you're going to stay this way forever.

Experience this often enough and it'll usually lead a traumatic dieter to abandon the entirety of their current weight management effort. And I don't blame them—who wants to live a life rife with self-loathing and guilt?

Instead of forbidding foods, traumatic dieters need to learn how to manage indulgences. You need to be able to utilize food for pleasure and comfort, and most important, you need to learn how to not feel guilty afterwards.

The good news is: doing so isn't impossible. It just requires you to outsmart evolution. If you've got any hope of conquering this vicious cycle, the first step will be to turn off your body's drive to eat. If you've done so well, and you've prevented hunger by means of well-timed meals and snacks, along with ensuring you've had at the very least your minimum amounts of calories and protein, you'll be able to start working on thoughtful reduction rather than relying on blind restriction.

Thoughtful reduction involves a two-question process. The first?

Is It Worth the Calories?

To answer the question fairly, knowing the calories is important. The fact is, some indulgences simply aren't worth their calories. By asking the question you'll eliminate a fair percentage. Take store-bought muffins, for instance. Maybe you order a Starbucks zucchini walnut muffin because you think at least then you're ordering something healthful. But would you order it if you realized it contained 490 calories? For many folks, that would be one-third of their total daily calories; it has nearly the calories of two Snickers bars and more than a McDonald's double cheeseburger. Is it so delicious that it's worth it? Personally, I've never met a store-bought muffin worth its calories.

The second question?

How Much of It Do I Need to Be Happy?

By asking this question you're avoiding the write-off situation where you pay no attention, eat the whole quantity in front of you, and then wind up feeling guilty about the amount of the food you consumed. But it doesn't have to be all or nothing. You can set yourself up to have as much of an indulgence as you need to really enjoy it, but not so much that you're stuffed to the gills by the time you're done. If chocolate is your thing, you might decide that one of those 100-calorie mini bars will do the trick. If it's cake, maybe a sliver rather than a big plateful? If it's ice cream, you might decide a measured half-cup would be enough to satisfy, rather than a blindly filled whole bowl. Or maybe you'll decide it's worth the full monty—a king-size bar, a 400-calorie slice, a pint of ice cream. What is important is that your decision's an informed one. Less isn't always more and sometimes life does—and frankly should—include a great many calories. But you owe it to yourself to be informed, and to be informed you need the numbers. Once informed, and with this question backing you up, you've got all the power.

Sometimes choosing the small portion will satisfy you. Sometimes it won't; when that's the case, simply ask the questions again and again until such time as you're content.

Remember, there are many variables that go into these decisions, and some days are worth more calories than others—birthdays, holidays, vacations, to name just a few. So the answers to these questions will actually vary day by day.

Ultimately, I want you to choose with your brain, not with your body, but again, you can do so only if you've taken your body out of the picture. If you're hungry, if you've missed meals, snacks, calories, or protein, your body and its years of painful evolution will almost certainly trump your brain.

WHEN TO INDULGE?

There may be a logical time this week. A birthday, a celebration, a holiday. But even if there's not, it's important to start including indulgences into your life right now. Indulgences shouldn't be in place of a regular meal or snack, unless the indulgence also satisfies your minimum calorie and protein requirements.

This part's crucial, especially for your first time: if you've traditionally been scared of losing control with your danger foods, you've got to try to indulge on a day when you've been especially well organized. It'll be a day when you've had all your meals and snacks, your timing's been great, and protein and calories are where you'd like them to be, not purposely on the lowest edge of your minimums. It's especially important for me to note: don't save up your calories so that you can have an indulgence, as that will tempt hunger and put you at much greater risk of losing control. Skimping on a few hundred calories during the day so that you can have some chocolate later leaves you open to consuming 500 calories' worth rather than a more tempered 150.

So what I want you to do is to choose a food that in your traumatic dieting effort past you'd have tried to avoid. But you don't need to flirt with disaster. If it's cookies, for instance, it may not be wise to bring home an entire bag, but certainly buying a cookie and truly enjoying it—that's important.

Make sure you've asked yourself your two questions before indulging, and if you'd like more, simply ask those questions again. Even if it leads you to consume a great many more calories than normal, don't worry. Remember that while it's certainly not a perfect formula, you can think of there being 3,500 calories in a pound, so even if you have 1,000 indulgent calories as you're getting your feet wet with thoughtful indulgence, it won't add up to even one-third of a pound.

While a few cookies now and again aren't going to sink your weight management efforts, not having them might.

End of Day Checklist

(If you've missed anything, restart Day 7 again tomorrow, and don't spend even a moment beating yourself up about it—life happens.)

- ☐ Your home-cooked foods were all weighed and measured
- ☐ Your food was completely diarized, nonjudgmentally, in real time—good, bad, and ugly, without artificial restrictions
- ☐ Your meals each contained at least one-fifth of your total daily recommended caloric aim and at least 20 grams of protein
- ☐ Your snacks each contained at least 150 calories and at least 10 grams of protein
- ☐ You set up reminders to help yourself remember when to eat
- ☐ You ate an additional 150 calories for every 45 minutes you exercised vigorously, either immediately before or after your workout
- ☐ You ate more if you were hungry
- ☐ You performed at least your toothbrush level of exercise
- ☐ You cooked all of your meals and snacks today
- ☐ You enjoyed a thoughtful dietary indulgence
- ☐ You asked constructive, not destructive, questions if things weren't going according to plan
- ☐ You recognized that your personal best is great
- ☐ You read tomorrow's daily plan and you're ready for it
- ☐ You found someone to eat out with tomorrow night for dinner, and if necessary made reservations
- ☐ You congratulated yourself on being 70 percent Reset

DAY 8: EAT OUT!

So you've got yourself organized, learned how to diarize, eliminated hunger, started to cook, learned how to think differently, added in some exercise, and enjoyed some indulgent food. Today you're going to learn how to eat out.

Start of Day Checklist
(If you aren't ready with all of these, repeat the prior day's program.)

- You're prepared to weigh and measure foods and record in real time
- You're prepared to eat on the clock
- You're prepared to eat even if you're not in the mood
- You're prepared to cook each and every meal and snack for the remaining week, except for dinner tonight
- You've packed your lunch and snacks for work today
- You're prepared with constructive questions to deal with potentially destructive circumstances
- You've got exercise shoes and comfortable clothes at the ready, and you have at least your toothbrush level of exercise planned
- You're prepared with the two questions you need to manage a thoughtful indulgence
- You've got a restaurant picked out for dinner, and if you need them, you've made reservations

DON'T SAVE YOUR CALORIES FOR DINNER

Enjoying a nice meal out at a restaurant with friends or family is one of life's simplest pleasures.

Celebratory meals, social meals, and required business meals—these are either unavoidable or nonnegotiable, and all should remain part of your life. The meals out you really ought to lose? The convenience meals out, the "because I don't feel like cooking" meals out, the "it's been a long day and I earned a reward" meals out.

So how do you manage your day of your dinner out? Do you skip breakfast? Cut the snacks? Skimp all day long? Is the goal to try to save up calories so you've got more room at dinner? While those might sound like intuitively great ideas, my experience has taught me that saving calories is the last thing you ought to do, as without a doubt, you'll end up overeating at dinner by more calories than you saved during the day. Remember, if you save up the calories, you're just going to switch on those 100 million years of hunger-satisfying evolution, and even if you try to be "good," and despite being hungry, choose a lower-calorie, healthier-choice meal, you are going to pay. Here the cost won't be calories, it'll be bitterness, as hunger affects the emotional interpretation of your meal. Order "healthy" when you're hungry and craving not-healthy and expect to be muttering under your breath about your *stupid diet.* If you regularly feel bitter about what you're "allowed" to eat in restaurants, that is a surefire way to ensure that eventually you'll be giving up on your healthy living strategies.

The healthiest lifestyle you can enjoy doesn't have to mean a food-as-fuel, exercise-as-life lifestyle. Life needs to include meals out, and tonight you're going to have one. First, let me give you some pointers and tips to help with your night.

PLAN AHEAD

It's easier than it used to be to plan your meal ahead now that many restaurants post calories and nutritional information online. Before you go out, given that you know where you're going, search online to see if you can find the menu's nutritional breakdown. Most fast-casual restaurants will share online, and if you can't find it, www.calorieking.com and www.myfitnesspal.com have compiled most chain restaurants' calorie listings.

If you do find calories posted, use them as just one decision-making variable. You shouldn't aim to automatically order the lowest-calorie item on the menu. You should aim to order the lowest-calorie item on the menu that you think you'll actually enjoy, and since our hankerings for foods change as the day progresses, it may be worth selecting a few options to choose from.

If you do find posted calories, when recording and considering them, I want you to add another 20 percent. The reason is that studies on the accuracy of posted restaurant calories suggest that they're far from perfectly accurate.[1] There have even been class action lawsuits launched against Applebee's, Chili's, On the Border, Macaroni Grill, and Weight Watchers following the laboratory evaluation of restaurant meals listed as being low in calories (and specially designed for WeightWatchers) when the results demonstrated markedly higher calories—sometimes more than double—than what was posted.

Additionally, the posted calories are the ones you might find in an idealized portion. Speaking with a fast-casual restaurant franchisee (he agreed to chat only if I promised not to mention his name or his restaurant's name), I asked him whether he thought his restaurant's posted calorie counts were accurate. Without hesitation he said "no" and explained that it was a matter of customer service. He told me that his instructions to his kitchen staff were to always err on the side of more rather than less: if there was any problem with the service, if the restaurant was busy and it took awhile to put in or make the order, if the plated food didn't look quite right, to simply plate more, as the larger portion would likely assuage the customer's frustration. What that means is that even if you look up the calories beforehand or at the point of purchase, in actuality the portion you receive might have even double the posted calories!

So what should you do if you don't find your planned restaurant's calories posted? Guess. Troll around those websites to look up comparable dishes, but this time, rather than add 20 percent to your estimate, add

---

THE "DOUBLE DOWN" PHENOMENON

As noted, restaurant calories are anything but intuitive, and to truly emphasize this point, I want to revisit the risks of eating out without considering calories by exploring common fast food fare and considering them in the context of the infamous KFC Double Down.

In case you don't remember, the Double Down was KFC's breadless offering that involved two fried chicken cutlets serving as the "bread" while the "sandwich" filling was cheese and bacon. The media went wild for the Double Down. Nutritionists the world over had nothing but scorn.

I was amazed. Sure, it's definitely shocking, but more from a yuck factor perspective than a nutritional one. Nutritionally, it sure is salty at 1,380 milligrams of sodium, but calorically it's a bit of a fast food yawn at 540 calories. That's basically a Big Mac with a tiny shake of salt on top.

What's important for people to understand is that the Double Down, when compared to many fast food options, is actually more typical than terrible. Want some perspective? Here are ten common fast food items, ranked by calories, that put the Double Down to shame, despite in many cases sounding like healthier options. This was by no means a difficult search, either. It took about 10 minutes, and had I bothered to explore items other than sandwiches I'd have found thousands of offerings (including salads) that while sounding healthy would have crushed the Double Down's (DD's) calorie totals.

10. Burger King Tendercrisp Chicken Sandwich on Artisan Bun
750 calories (1.4DDs), 1,560 mg sodium ▸

9. Dunkin' Donuts Tuna Melt Sandwich
   770 calories (1.4 DDs), 1,560 mg sodium

8. Au Bon Pain Southwest Tuna Wrap
   800 calories (1.5 DDs), 1,190 mg sodium

7. A&W Double Grandma Burger
   800 calories (1.5 DDs), 910 mg sodium

6. Arby's Roast Turkey Ranch and Bacon Sandwich
   800 calories (1.5 DDs), 2,200 mg sodium

5. Ruby Tuesday Avocado Turkey Burger
   968 calories (1.8 DDs), 1,601 mg sodium

4. Dairy Queen ½-pound Flamethrower Burger
   1,000 calories (1.9 DDs), 1,610 mg sodium

3. Boston's The Gourmet Pizza's Boston Cheeseburger Sandwich
   1,170 calories (2.1 DDs) 1,750 mg sodium

2. Applebee's Quesadilla Burger
   1,420 calories (2.6 DDs), 3,630 mg sodium

1. Quiznos Large Tuna Melt Sub
   1,460 calories (2.7 DDs), 1,780 mg sodium

And so the lesson is that calories are anything but intuitive. Prior to going out, exploring nutritional information may be eye-opening and may guide ordering—but don't forget, that information may still be inaccurate, and consequently I recommend adding 20 percent to posted fast food calories and 40 percent to posted fast-casual calories. ⊚

40 percent. Again, those numbers aren't meant to depress you or discourage you from ordering a meal that you'll really enjoy; they're just there to help you in your decision making.

PRE-EAT

Most of us, when we go out for dinner, tend to start and finish later than if we were cooking for ourselves. I'll often encourage people to have *an extra snack* just before they head out to dinner, so that when they finally do sit down to order, their brains can choose their best options from the menu without being pushed around by their bodies. If an extra 150-calorie snack is enough to help you avoid a 600-calorie appetizer, or leave behind some of your 1,200-calorie main course, well, that's a very fair trade.

I'll give you an example of how I use pre-eating in my life. There's this wing place. It's in Toronto and it's called The Bistro on Avenue, and I've been going there since I was around 16 years old. It's this great hole in the wall and the wings are just phenomenal. There are two sizes of wings at The Bistro, regular and large. I figure that before I moved to Ottawa at the age of 26, I must have gone to The Bistro for wings at least 150 times, and never once did I order a regular size. Fast-forward to my thirties. The Bistro had franchised and lo and behold, they arrived in Ottawa with the franchise name St. Louis. Of course, by now I'd learned a bit about nutrition and health, and while wings weren't eliminated from my lifestyle, they were downgraded to just a few times a year.

Before I went, I decided to try to calculate the calories in their portions. My best guess was that their large basket of wings, fries, and garlic dipping sauce clocked in at around 4,000 calories, while their regular at half the size ran nearer to 2,000. Going there now, the day a visit is planned I go out of my way to eat really well. I'll have all my meals and snacks, and often eat an extra 300 to 600 calories of snacks during the afternoon leading up to my night out. Having done so, I can comfortably sit down, order the regular size, and not feel shortchanged or anxious that I won't be satisfied. Spending 300 to 600 calories to save 2,000? Well, that's a pretty fair trade and a great investment.

Those few times a year that I go for my wings fix, so long as I've pre-eaten, my calories clock in somewhere around 3,500. That's still less than I'd have in total if I skipped every single meal and snack throughout my day and just showed up at St. Louis' ravenous for dinner. I'd have the

4,000 calories in the large, and tack on at least two drafts and now I'm up at close to 4,400 calories, 900 higher than my pre-eating day, which still included some beer and wings.

Remember, it's not about sticking your calorie landing like a gymnast. I don't need or want you to think that you're never, ever allowed to exceed your caloric aims. Instead, it's about the smallest number of calories you need to enjoy your day, even if the smallest number is higher than what you burn. From time to time, you're going to overspend, and that's okay.

Now, I'm not saying you should take this as an invitation to hit a wing joint every night. All I'm saying is that if you plan ahead and pre-eat, you'll be able to hang on to control over your decisions and navigate any menu comfortably; the end result will be that you will eat fewer total calories than you would trying to save them up.

OTHER COMMON EATING OUT CONSIDERATIONS

Post Drink

If you enjoy alcohol, avoiding the pre-dinner drink might help your night go a tad smoother. Alcohol is an appetite stimulant; it also affects decision making and tends to dissolve resolve. When the waitstaff shows up before you've ordered and asks you if you'd like a drink before ordering, resist. And if alcohol must be part of your night, start in on it only after dinner is served.

Don't Be Shy

Waitstaff welcome the opportunity to answer questions and entertain requests, because doing so will likely lead to a higher tip at the end of the night. So don't hesitate to ask questions and to get creative if you're not sure about what your best menu option is. While you can order off the kids' menu or have an appetizer as your main course, you can also just as easily ask for some modifications to your menu option—ask your server to have the kitchen plate only half a portion, or see if they can't whip up an off-the-menu selection for you. You're the customer. You need never feel shy about ensuring your purchase fits your needs and desires.

Skip the Doggy Bag

Remember the story I told you about the reality show contestant whose beet salad appetizer and fish main course had more than 2,000 calories?

So let's say she was doing the pretty common dieting practice of eating only half her meal. She'd still be downing an astounding 1,050 for that meal (not including beverage or dessert).

And if she got a doggy bag, she'd be doing it again for lunch.

I get it. I'm thrifty, too, and I feel like I ought to bring food home if I've already paid for it. But really, is it worth the calories?

Sometimes the answer to that question is going to be yes, absolutely; if it's an awesome meal, by all means, have it again for lunch! Calories be damned, it's your choice to enjoy that food the second time around. But if it's just a mediocre meal, do yourself a favor—leave those calories behind at the restaurant.

Use Your Napkin

I'm not talking about manners. What I'm talking about is something you do, I do, and everyone does. If there's still food on your plate and it's sitting in front of you waiting for the waitstaff to clear it away, you're going to keep pecking at it.

What I'll do to stop myself from mindlessly going back for more is fairly simple. As soon as I've decided I've had enough, I take the napkin out of my lap, wipe my mouth with it, and place it over my food. By covering up the plate of food staring at me, I'm far less likely to go digging for those mindless calories.

AN EATING OUT RULE OF THUMB

Back in the 1970s we used to spend just over 30 percent of our food dollars on meals purchased outside the home. Nowadays we're around the 50 percent mark. There's no doubt that society's increased frequency of meals out is contributing to our struggles with weight. Chances are, if you're over the age of 40 and you think back to when you were a kid, I'm guessing meals out were an incredibly rare event, whereas in my office today, I'm less likely to meet someone who's eating out less than once a week than I am to meet someone eating out daily.

While it's probably not a mathematical truth, here's a sobering concept that I find really lays bare the reality of the situation: every day that you're eating a meal out is a day that you're not likely to lose weight. Sure, there are lower-calorie options on many menus, but most options, even ones that sound healthful, are usually markedly higher in calories than anyone would ever guess—and probably also higher in calories and less healthful than what you would have made for yourself at home.

FAST FOOD VERSUS SIT DOWN

You know, I think fast food gets a bad rap. That's not to say fast food's a healthy choice, one that I'd recommend you make regularly, but there are a great many folks out there who think that they're far better off nutritionally and calorically hitting a so-called sit-down restaurant rather than a fast food one.

Nutritionally, there might be an argument to make in favor of sit down, but of course that's only if you go out of your way to choose nutritious options, which most of us probably don't.

Calorically, I'm guessing fast food wins more often than not, and it wins for two reasons. First, it's basically made by machines. Not to say that people aren't involved, but it's more of an assembly line than a kitchen, and as mentioned earlier, once people get involved in cooking and plating, calories tend to go up higher than you might expect. Second, in a fast food restaurant there aren't any bread baskets, usually there aren't appetizers, rarely are they licensed to serve alcohol, and given the options, you might be less likely to order up dessert.

I'm not suggesting you head out to fast food joints regularly, but I definitely don't want you thinking that doing so is somehow riskier than a sit-down establishment. ⊚

I've had patients tell me that their meals out are safe, but given the inaccuracy of posted calories, the fact that a restaurant's or cafeteria's job is to make food taste good, and the fact that calories make food taste good, I'm skeptical.

Eat out more than once or twice a week and losing weight that week's going to be a challenge. Eat out more than three times a week and fair or not, you very well might end up gaining—and that'd be true even if the rest of your week was beautifully managed.

I ATE OUT LAST NIGHT AND GAINED TWO POUNDS

I want to say one more thing about eating out in restaurants.

While it's true restaurant meals can contain astounding numbers of calories, if you step on the scale the next morning and you're two pounds heavier than the morning before, the scale's measuring something other than your real weight. The most likely culprit is water retention consequent to having a great deal more sodium in your dinner than you normally do at home.

As mentioned earlier, people aren't walking mathematical formulae, and they gain and lose different amounts of weight for the same degree of excess or restriction, but the fact remains that people cannot create energy, and weight is simply stored energy. For you to gain two actual pounds in a night would require at *the very least* the consumption of 7,000 additional calories, calories above and beyond the calories you normally burn in a day. I'm pretty sure you didn't eat 7,000 calories for dinner. To do so would involve eating three racks of ribs with two large servings of fries, or an 8-pound steak, or 20 pieces of KFC, or four medium pepperoni pizzas. ⊙

End of Day Checklist
(If you've missed anything, restart Day 8 again tomorrow, and don't spend even a moment beating yourself up about it—life happens.)

☐ Your home-cooked foods were all weighed and measured

☐ Your food was completely diarized, nonjudgmentally, in real time—good, bad, and ugly, without artificial restrictions

☐ Your meals each contained at least one-fifth of your total daily recommended caloric aim and at least 20 grams of protein

☐ Your snacks each contained at least 150 calories and at least 10 grams of protein

☐ You set up reminders to help yourself remember when to eat

☐ You ate an additional 150 calories for every 45 minutes you exercised vigorously, either immediately before or after your workout

☐ You ate more if you were hungry

☐ You performed at least your toothbrush level of exercise

☐ You cooked all of your meals and snacks today other than dinner

☐ You ate out thoughtfully and without guilt, having planned and pre-eaten

☐ You asked constructive, not destructive, questions if things weren't going according to plan

☐ You recognized that your personal best is great

☐ You read tomorrow's daily plan and you're ready for it

☐ You congratulated yourself on being 80 percent Reset

DAY 9: SET GOALS!

S o you've got yourself organized, learned how to diarize, eliminated hunger, started to cook, learned how to think differently, added in some exercise, enjoyed some indulgent food, and eaten out. Today you're going to learn how to set some truly useful goals.

Start of Day Checklist
(If you aren't ready with all of these, repeat your prior day's program.)

- You're prepared to weigh and measure foods and record in real time
- You're prepared to eat on the clock
- You're prepared to eat even if you're not in the mood
- You're prepared to cook each and every meal and snack for the remaining week
- You've packed your lunch and snacks for work today
- You're prepared with constructive questions to deal with potentially destructive circumstances
- You've got exercise shoes and comfortable clothes at the ready, and you have at least your toothbrush level of exercise planned
- You have some index cards or a notepad that you can write on, and a pen to write with, and three (just three) minutes alone set aside this morning, before work, for a quick mental exercise

Life is anything but a straight line, and this journey isn't going to be one, either. Whether you're doing this to break free of diet-centricity, to maintain a weight you're comfortable with, or to lose further, there are going to be days, weeks, and potentially even months when life trumps your best intentions.

That doesn't mean you can't help yourself. Here are some straightforward tips and techniques to try to troubleshoot struggle. Practicing them when the going's good will help you to employ them when it's not. Remember, changes—even straightforward changes—can be difficult to remember to do. These techniques are designed to help you remember a way of living that your life won't inherently remind you to do.

VISUALIZATION

Don't groan. It may seem hokey, but there's likely not a professional athlete on the planet who doesn't use visualizations to help them play at the top of their game.

You can use them, too, and I promise they won't take long.

Let's say you're having a difficult time remembering to use your food diary. Here's an easy visualization exercise you can employ that takes all of 30 seconds, a few times a day.

In the morning when you've got one minute to yourself, take a piece of paper about the size of an index card or a small notepad and on it write, in first-person present tense:

Every time I eat, I pull out my food diary and record what I've eaten.

Now that you've written it, if you're brave enough, I want you to read it out loud. After you've read it once or twice with conviction, I want you to close your eyes and picture yourself at your meals and snacks throughout the day. Put as much detail in it as possible. Include what you're wearing. Try to imagine exactly where you'll be. Add in thoughts about the sounds, smells, and lighting around you. Then visualize yourself pulling out the snack or meal you've already planned for the day, see yourself eating your meal or snack, and as soon as you've finished, visualize yourself pulling out your food diary and your pen (or smartphone, or keyboard), writing it down, and putting your diary away. You should also imagine the sense of pride you'll feel for following through. I want you to spend at least 30 seconds visualizing diarizing each meal and snack, which means this whole exercise should take no more than two and a half minutes. While some dedicated moments may work best, if you're truly pressed for time, multitask it. Make a habit out of visualizing at preset times, such as when brushing your teeth, while waiting for your toaster to pop, or when you're stuck at a red light.

The first few times you try, the detail won't be great and it may feel like an odd thing to do, but as you get more experienced in visualizing, you'll be able to add more and more detail. Basically, you're training your mind to become an artist, a painter, and while your strokes might start out as rough and halting, unlike with real painting it doesn't take too much practice before you'll get great. Once you're great, the time you'll need may well go down to where just 10 seconds per meal or snack will suffice.

This type of visualization exercise can be used for any behavior you're trying to cultivate. Just make sure that when you write on your piece of paper, you always make it personal by using the word "I," and always write in present tense (therefore, don't write "I will"; write, "I always").

I always walk for ten minutes when I come home from work.
I always check the fridge and the freezer to see what's on hand before I order in take-out.
I always remember to snack in between meals.

Feel free to use as many different visualizations per day as you think will help.

SET A BETTER WEIGHT GOAL

Most traumatic dieters will see numbers as their ultimate goal. They want to reach their "ideal" weight, or fit into a particular clothing size, or at the very least, reach some specific number on a scale.

Numbers are truly lousy goals, and I'd like to help you to set better ones.

When it comes to the intersection of healthy lifestyle and healthy weight, there are really only two primary goals to set. The first would be to eat the smallest number of calories you need to like your life, and the second would be to exercise as much as you can enjoy.

Notice that there's pleasure associated with both goals. Sure, you'd be able to tolerate less food and more exercise, but a lifestyle that's only tolerable isn't likely to be a lifestyle you're going to sustain. The simple fact is that there comes a point beyond which you truly shouldn't eat less, because if you did it would lead you to feel hungry, feel unwell, or feel as if your life is abnormal. Normal life includes occasional food for comfort and food for celebration, and there's no such thing as an always forbidden food.

Similarly, there comes a point beyond which you shouldn't exercise more because if you did you'd run out of time, run out of energy, hurt yourself, or just hate it—if any of those things happened, you'd likely quit.

As far as living a long-term lifestyle rather than a short-term diet goes, if you can't happily eat less, you're not going to eat less, and if you can't happily exercise more, you're not going to exercise more.

That's why your goal is to live the healthiest life you can enjoy, not the healthiest life you can tolerate, and whatever weight you reach once you're living that life, well, remember, that's what I would refer to as your "best weight."

GET THERE WITH BEHAVIOR GOALS

If you get a Visa bill that's higher than you'd like, do you simply wish it lower for the next month, or might you try to adjust your spending? The Visa total—that's the consequence of your spending, which is the cause of your high bill. If you'd like to change next month's Visa total, then you'll probably have to tackle next month's spending. Your weight isn't any different. Your weight is the consequence of many factors, and while there are definitely many causes beyond your control (genetics, job requirements, stress, travel, caring for kids/parents, an obesogenic environment, etc.), there are some weight contributors that are modifiable. Therefore, rather than set numbered weight goals, it's much wiser to set goals based on those.

One of the primary reasons for goal setting is for you to be proud of yourself. Pride, despite it being one of the traditional seven deadly sins, is also a very powerful positive emotion. It's much easier to move forward with behavior changes if you're proud of yourself than if you always beat yourself up. Ensuring that you've got achievable goals is one way to ensure you can build some positive emotion into your efforts.

HOW TO SET A SMART GOAL

Setting achievable goals is crucial, and consequently goals need to reflect SMART principles: your goals need to be Specific, Measureable, Attainable, Relevant, and Time bound.

Put another way, you need to choose goals that are achievable in a timely manner and measurable in terms of success. "Exercising more" would be an example of an un-SMART goal, whereas "going for a 10-minute walk every weekday morning before breakfast" is a SMART one.

The more specific you can make your goal, the better. Make sure, too, that the goal has the "how" in it.

Here are a few "eat healthier" examples:

Before I put anything in my supermarket cart, I will look at the food label.

I will put together a shopping list before each and every supermarket visit.

On Sunday mornings, after breakfast, I will find a new healthy recipe to cook, put together a shopping list for it on the spot, schedule a day for shopping, and plan my night for cooking.

Here are a few weight management examples:

I'm going to keep a food diary for at least a month to start looking for calories I can lose without missing them.

I'm going to eat every two and a half to three and a half hours and will set alarms and reminders to help me do it.

I'm going to include protein in every meal and snack to minimize hunger.

I'm going to eat within half an hour of waking and have at least 350 calories for breakfast.

If you're going to set a goal, don't forget the specifics and the hows. Also, keep it simple, as the more complicated or dramatic the goal, the tougher it'll be to gather those small victories.

If you're looking to set up some goals, following you'll find a list of examples of healthy living goal-setting targets ripe for SMARTifying. Once you've come up with some SMART goals, find somewhere to keep track of them. Every week, or perhaps even every day, pull them out and review. Sometimes goals you thought were SMART may turn out to be only SMRT (missing the attainable part) and consequently you won't be able to follow through. When that happens, try to think of a way to shrink your goal. For example, maybe your goal was 20 minutes every morning on the treadmill before breakfast. Switch it to five and see how you do.

Examples of healthy living goals that you can SMARTify, which have an impact on weight, may include:

- Learning how to cook healthy meals from real food staples rather than ordering in, taking out, or reheating a box.
- Brown-bagging your lunches.
- Insisting on a few moments of *you* time every day. Time you might use to take a brief walk, self-reflect, positively affirm, and recharge. You and I both know that while it's certainly important to take care of your family, always putting them ahead of yourself doesn't teach them the importance of self-care, and also doesn't allow you

to nurture yourself—and that makes it more difficult to truly care for them.

- Working up to being able to walk a certain distance or at a certain speed, or being able to keep up with your children or grandchildren.
- Being able to walk up a flight or two of stairs without feeling winded.
- Participating in a community race.
- Taking a moment here and there to tell your loved ones how much you love and appreciate them. Healthy lives definitely benefit from healthy relationships.
- Being proud of yourself and taking the time to appreciate your personal victories. Sure, other people may be better at healthy living than you (Lord knows many are better than me), maybe it comes more easily to other people, but the fact is, you are taking the steps you need to take to feel good about your life. And recognizing that isn't a bad thing. In fact, it's empowering, as it'll provide you with ample opportunities to take some time to reflect not on your failures, but rather on your successes.
- Being comfortable in your own skin and not caring what others think.

Some goals may be related to weight, but not to a specific amount of loss. Those goals may include:

- Being able to comfortably cross your legs, tie your shoes, or get up from the floor gracefully.
- Being able to fit in smaller-size clothing that you may have hanging around from earlier years.
- Being able to resume playing a sport you used to enjoy.
- Coming off or reducing some medications for weight-related conditions.
- Shopping off the rack in a "regular" store.

End of Day Checklist

(If you've missed anything, restart Day 9 again tomorrow, and don't spend even a moment beating yourself up about it—life happens.)

- [ ] Your home-cooked foods were all weighed and measured
- [ ] Your food was completely diarized, nonjudgmentally, in real time—good, bad, and ugly, without artificial restrictions
- [ ] Your meals each contained at least one-fifth of your total daily recommended caloric aim and at least 20 grams of protein
- [ ] Your snacks each contained at least 150 calories and at least 10 grams of protein
- [ ] You set up reminders to help yourself remember when to eat
- [ ] You ate an additional 150 calories for every 45 minutes you exercised vigorously, either immediately before or after your workout
- [ ] You ate more if you were hungry
- [ ] You performed at least your toothbrush level of exercise
- [ ] You cooked all of your meals and snacks today
- [ ] You asked constructive, not destructive, questions if things weren't going according to plan
- [ ] You recognized that your personal best is great
- [ ] You practiced visualizing your success
- [ ] You set some SMART goals
- [ ] You read tomorrow's daily plan and you're ready for it
- [ ] You congratulated yourself on being 90 percent Reset

DAY 10: TROUBLESHOOT AND MOVE FORWARD!

So you've got yourself organized, learned how to diarize, eliminated hunger, started to cook, learned how to think differently, added in some exercise, enjoyed some indulgent food, eaten out, and set useful goals. Today you're going to learn how to take what you've learned and pay it forward for the rest of your life.

Start of Day Checklist
(If you aren't ready with all of these, repeat the prior day's program.)

- You're prepared to weigh and measure foods and record in real time
- You're prepared to eat on the clock
- You're prepared to eat even if you're not in the mood
- You're prepared to cook each and every meal and snack from now on (well, most of them, anyway)
- You've packed your lunch and snacks for work today
- You're prepared with constructive questions to deal with potentially destructive circumstances
- You've got exercise shoes and comfortable clothes at the ready, and you have at least your toothbrush level of exercise planned
- You've got your morning visualizations ready
- You've set and can recall your SMART goals

It's the last day of your Reset. You've spent the past nine days exploring the impact of organization on choice and of thoughtfulness on attitude. My hope is that by being carefully organized, you've managed to turn off your body's drive to eat and that with those urges quieted, you've been able to follow through with healthier choices without it being a fight. By rethinking goals, you'll have recognized that the scale is not the arbiter of success and that your personal best is the only goal worth setting—and that your personal best actually changes day by day.

It's important to remember that this is a journey. It's taken you much longer than 10 days to get to this point in your life, and it's going to take you much longer than 10 days to truly leave.

Unlike traumatic dieting, however, this is only going to get easier with time. With traumatic dieting, life gets more difficult. The restrictions and the fights with cravings and hunger amplify over time, until eventually you crash. This approach is different. This approach relies on organization and thinking—both of which will get easier, not more difficult. The more often you work on something's organization, the easier it will become to organize, and eventually, habits will form.

But of course there will be some roadblocks and hurdles along the way:

HEAD OFF THE MOST COMMON ROADBLOCKS

"I'm too busy to . . ."

I'd say that's the roadblock I hear more frequently than any other in my office, and honestly, it should be the least likely to trip you up.

While I certainly believe that people are busy, I also know that if you're serious about trying to get a handle on things, you'll be able to find the 15 to 30 minutes a day you need to help in your lifestyle's restructuring. If you feel you honestly don't have, can't find, or can't spare 15 to 30 minutes, it might be worth exploring the reasons why.

To help, let's go through some "too busy's."

Too Busy to Cook
I covered this bit on Day 4, but it's important enough to re-review.

- Ensure that you've got grocery shopping as a scheduled, recurrent weekly event.
- Next, ensure that your freezer has some emergency meals.
- Lastly, when you do cook, remember to cook lots.

As a very last resort, explore your Yellow Pages or the Internet to look for a company that makes fresh, calorie-controlled meals and delivers them to your home. I call this a last resort both because of the expense, and because as a natural born skeptic, I tend not to trust the calorie calculations of others, especially others who stand to profit from you thinking *this tastes too good to have only this many calories* and may benefit from underreporting.

Too Busy to Snack

I know I'm a bit of a broken record, but for many of my patients, healthy, protein-inclusive snacking is a true turning point behavior and so I want to review some common barriers.

Snacking is probably the preemptive eating behavior that people struggle with the most. More often than not it's because people feel that they are simply too busy to snack, when really they're just too busy to remember to. Don't forget to set up reminders to help:

At home: Kitchen timers, oven timers, microwave timers, spouses, partners, and children

At the office: Outlook reminders

Out and about: Smartphone or cell phone alarms (to which you can assign a specific ringtone), free online text messaging services such as www.ohdontforget.com, or calendar reminders (Google calendars can be trained to do that)

Remember, too, snacking need not take a long time, and if you're always feeling pressured for time with your snacks, make sure that you're choosing quick options.

Too Busy to Record

This one I hear a lot, but I never buy it. If you've got time to eat, you've got time to record what you've eaten. It takes at most 30 seconds to record even the largest meal (and remember, you can look the calories up later).

Don't forget you can use shorthand. If you're a creature of habit and you have only one or two breakfasts or snacks every day, then simply write them as B1, B2, S1, and S2 to keep track. Those few milliseconds of scribbling really do have tremendous power, and it'd be a huge shame for you to lose that advantage.

Often the folks who report they're too busy to record are the folks who are having the most difficult time letting go of the notion that their food diaries are judges and juries. Always keep in mind that the record is there simply to guide future dietary decisions, not to judge those that are past, and that your food diary, like mine, definitely won't be full of perfect choices.

There may be circumstances here and there, and from time to time, that preclude your best efforts and strategies. The secret then is just to pick up where you left off as soon as life allows.

Too Busy to Exercise

If you have a favorite television show that you watch regularly, then clearly you're not too busy to exercise, you're simply choosing not to.

I'm not trying to get all preachy here—sometimes you may well be too stressed, too tired, or too worn out to exercise, and would rather just collapse in a heap in front of the television than head out in the rain or cold for a walk.

Folks who think they're too busy to exercise should really focus on what I referred to earlier in the book as "functional exercise"—the stuff you've got to do anyway that doesn't feel like exercise.

I also recommend that they truly work on figuring out their "tooth-brush levels" of exercise, and then schedule them in specifically, as often the folks who feel they're too busy for exercise are the folks who are still clinging to the notion that exercise needs to be of lengthy duration and high intensity to count.

MY 10 CARDINAL RULES

If you get stuck in a funk of feeling overwhelmed with this, let me break down Reset's 10 most basic principles. If you're truly struggling, your job is to focus on these 10 points to pull yourself back together. There are no maximums here, just minimums, meaning the only limits to set for yourself are to ensure you eat enough of something, rather than stress out over trying not to have too much.

While there are dozens of elements to a healthy, nontraumatic lifestyle, some elements are more important to success than others. If I had to boil it down to just 10 rules, it would be these. Get these back under control, and everything else ought to fall back into place:

1. Eat breakfast within 60 minutes of waking up.
2. Eat every two and a half to three and a half hours.
3. Ensure that your meals have a bare minimum of one-fifth of your daily *non–weight loss* calorie needs.
4. Ensure that your snacks have a bare minimum of 150 calories.
5. Ensure that each meal contains 20 or more grams of protein and each snack 10 or more grams.
6. Limit refined/processed foods to the smallest amounts you need to be happy.
7. Drink only as many calories as you need to enjoy your life (that means minimize juice, alcohol, sugared beverages, milk, etc.).
8. Exercise for 45 minutes or less, and all you need is water. Exercise vigorously for more than 45 minutes, and add 150 calories per 45-minute block, to be consumed immediately before or immediately after exercise.
9. There should be no such thing as a forbidden food.
10. Always, always, always consider the calories of your dietary decisions in the same manner you consider price tags with your purchases.

Once you feel like you're on solid ground again, then you can focus on fine-tuning calories and other behaviors.

End of Day Checklist
(If you've missed anything, restart Day 10 again tomorrow, and don't spend even a moment beating yourself up about it—life happens.)

- ☐ Your home-cooked foods were all weighed and measured
- ☐ Your food was completely diarized, nonjudgmentally, in real time—good, bad, and ugly, without artificial restrictions
- ☐ Your meals each contained at least one-fifth of your total daily recommended caloric aim and at least 20 grams of protein
- ☐ Your snacks each contained at least 150 calories and at least 10 grams of protein
- ☐ You set up reminders to help yourself remember when to eat
- ☐ You ate an additional 150 calories for every 45 minutes you exercised vigorously, either immediately before or after your workout
- ☐ You ate more if you were hungry
- ☐ You performed at least your toothbrush level of exercise
- ☐ You cooked all of your meals and snacks today
- ☐ You asked constructive, not destructive, questions if things weren't going according to plan
- ☐ You recognized that your personal best is great
- ☐ You practiced visualizing your success
- ☐ You set some SMART goals
- ☐ You congratulated yourself on being 100 percent Reset
- ☐ You realize that success isn't about sacrifice, starvation, or struggle, but rather about lifelong planning, organizing, and thoughtfulness, and that those in turn get easier, not more difficult, with time

POST RESET

Now that you're comfortably Reset, it's time to move forward. By definition a *reset* suggests a new start, and by using the principles you've learned these past 10 days, you're now ready for the next steps.

Long-term success requires consistency, and it's the principles you've learned, the tools you've gathered, and the attitudes you've cultivated these past 10 days that will set you off on a lifelong journey. Ten days isn't sufficient to erase the scars of a lifetime of traumatic dieting, nor is it enough time to lose a dramatic amount of weight. There's also no doubt that life's adventures will also occasionally blow you off course. Learning how to pick yourself up and dust yourself off is crucial. So, too, is never wavering from the belief that true success comes from recognizing your personal best as great, and not from some idealized societal or medical number–based goal.

While these first 10 days may have provided you with a taste of life beyond traumatic dieting, there's more I'd like to share with you—some basics about nutrition, a discussion of the impact of different medications and medical problems, an explanation of both pharmacologic and surgical weight management considerations, some of my favorite recipes, and perhaps most important, a discussion of how these principles can be applied to any diet or weight management program you might choose to consider.

The Recovery

Ten days into the rest of your life and what have you learned?

You've learned that organization is more important than deprivation; that willpower is the absence of hunger; that kitchens have a greater impact on weight than spin classes; that thinking and planning are more important to weight management than sacrifice and suffering; that perfection's a terrible goal; that your personal best is great; and that real life includes chocolate. In a sense, these past 10 days you've built and fortified your life's new food foundation. Now it's time to start building your new home.

But remember, it's a custom home you're building. One of the biggest problems with modern dieting theory is the belief that there is only one right way to go. Rather than embrace the diversity of people, palates, cultures, and tastes, modern-day dieting dumbs us down to dietary automatons who are given rules about what we can and can't eat, and who are told that breaking those rules is akin to religious sinning. The secret to long-term success with weight management is actually liking your life, because regardless of how much weight you might lose on a particular dietary approach, if you don't actually like your life while you're losing, you'll eventually head back to the life (and weight) you were living before you lost.

Remember, too, that life's not a straight line and that there will be circumstances that will have an impact on your personal bests. I want to provide you with as many strategies as possible to get you through some of real life's most common hiccups—things like vacations, conferences, illnesses, religious holidays, celebrations, and sorrows—as learning to roll with these punches is crucial to your long-term success. I'll even cover how to use your bathroom scale safely, as using it the wrong way can break even the most thoughtful dieter. All of this just goes to show you that it's just not as simple as "eat less, move more" when it comes to weight management or to recovering from traumatic dieting.

I'm going to break this information down into sections: Diet, Live, Eat, Move, Think, Weigh, Heal, and Parent.

- In *Diet,* we'll go over how you can use your Reset principles to Reset any diet or program of your choosing.
- In *Live,* we'll go over some skills and tricks for vacations, conferences, and weekends, as well as how to choose a better drink and how to set actually useful New Year's resolutions.
- In *Eat,* we'll explore many more of the nuances of a healthy relationship with food, including mindless eating, the surprising caloric difference between processed and whole foods, portion paralysis, and how to turn off your indulgence autopilots.
- In *Move,* we'll revisit exercise and explore easy ways to encourage yourself to add in more exercise, as well as weigh in on whether *The Biggest Loser*'s approach is a sound one.
- In *Think,* we'll review the means you might use to change your internal sound tracks; consider how to deal with food cops and food pushers; understand food addiction; contemplate when it might actually be worthwhile to suffer; and look at how you're actually going to maintain your new habits.
- In *Weigh,* we'll spend some time getting to know your scale and cover topics such as scale addiction, scale seduction, and scale avoidance, as well as explore scale holidays and whether there's really such a thing as the dreaded "plateau."
- In *Heal,* we'll discuss the impact different medications and medical conditions have on weight, alternatives to common medications that cause weight gain, and the realities of weight loss surgery, weight loss medications, and over-the-counter supplements.
- In *Parent,* we'll touch on how to craft a healthy home, how to eat during pregnancy, how the style you use to feed your children matters, and how to set up your kids for a lifetime of success.

RESET ANY DIET

It's important for you to know how you can use the Reset principles to reset any diet. While Reset's principles can be used as a stand-alone means to manage weight, they can also work alongside a particular diet plan or program. In fact, there's almost no diet or program that can't be Reset. Equally good news: just like everything else in life, when it comes to what's the best diet, there are different strokes for different folks. But what does *best* mean when it comes to a "best" diet? Does *best* mean the healthiest, or does *best* mean the most effective for weight management?

WHAT'S THE HEALTHIEST DIET?

I'd rather pose another question. If there were truly a "healthiest" diet, would that make following it any easier? Let's say low-carb was truly the way to go for health. Or perhaps veganism or macrobiotic vegetarianism. Or maybe a particular paleo advocate's approach. Or even the exceedingly low-fat plan advocated by Dean Ornish. Would knowing that a specific diet conferred the greatest health or weight management benefits ever outweigh the simple fact that if you don't happen to like what you're eating while on it, you'll probably not keep eating that way?

Personally, I don't think so, and that's why I'm going to refrain from getting into the nitty-gritty science of various dietary methodologies and theories and stick with what I know to be an incontrovertible fact: you have to like that way you're eating if you're going to eat that way forever.

There are pros and cons to virtually every dietary plan, whether it's low-carb, low-fat, vegan, Mediterranean, DASH, paleo, ancestral, fasting, or clean. There are health benefits to each and every one. You should know, too, that science isn't anywhere near being able to declare one diet the true health winner, and chances are it never will be. So I'll leave it to the various nutrition gurus and diet champions to duke it out, but ultimately, I'm guessing that every one of them would agree that if you don't want to get caught up in the minutiae of trying to stick perfectly to any one approach, then going to restaurants far less often, using fewer boxes in your meal preparations, and performing far more in the way of from-scratch transformations of whole food ingredients would go an extremely long way toward improving your health and managing your weight.

RESETTING LOW-CARB DIETS (ATKINS, 17 DAY, DUKAN, WHEAT BELLY, SOUTH BEACH)

Low-carb diets have been around for a long time. One of the best-selling British books of the 19th century was in fact a low-carb diet, written in 1863 by William Banting. Banting was a formerly obese carpenter and undertaker, and his book, *Letter on Corpulence Addressed to the Public*, might be fairly described as the first diet book blockbuster. It wasn't a book by today's standard—probably better described as a long pamphlet—but as mentioned earlier, it was so widely read that according to the Weston Price Foundation (a low-carb proponent group), people used the term *banting* in place of *dieting*.[1] Banting's description of his strategy was straightforward:

> Bread, butter, milk, sugar, beer, and potatoes, which had been the main (and, I thought, innocent) elements of my subsistence, or at all events they had for many years been adopted freely.
>
> These, said my excellent adviser, contain starch and saccharine matter, tending to create fat, and should be avoided altogether.[2]

That description—eliminating carbohydrates, sugars, and simple starches—while tweaked and massaged by different low-carb diets, is their underlying commonality. Interestingly, then, just as now, many doctors looked down their noses at Banting's suggestions, but then, just as now, those doctors probably needn't have worried. Having met many patients who stopped their low-carb diets because their physicians or friends convinced them the diets were unhealthy, it's probably in order to take a quick look at what tends to worry people about them.

Many opponents to low-carb diets worry a great deal about their supposed risks. They worry that eating so much dietary fat (it follows that if there are only three macronutrient categories—fats, proteins, and carbohydrates—when you cut out carbs, you'll eat more fats) will lead to hardening of the arteries and other medical complications. I honestly think those folks are out to a low-fat lunch. Simply put, dietary fats have been wrongly vilified by the medical community for decades. Three recent meta-analyses of the medical literature around saturated fat consumption and its impact on death and cardiovascular disease have all independently exonerated saturated fat as something you need to inherently worry about.[3] While there are those out there who still debate the impact of different types of fats, the simplest way to look at our current evidence-based consensus on fat is:

- Artificially made trans-fats are bad and should be avoided.
- Saturated fats (mainly found in meats and dairy products) aren't inherently nutritionally evil, and you can enjoy them within calorie limits.
- Unsaturated fats (found in fish, nuts, and certain oils, such as olive) probably confer some health benefits, and you might want to try to increase them in your diets.

So now that hopefully, you're no longer worried about saturated fats, I should also point out that studies done on low-carb diets have also shown them to be safe, at least in the short run (studies up to two years, for instance), and I don't think there's any good medical evidence or reasoning right now to suggest that they wouldn't be safe in the long run, either.

As far as resetting a low-carb diet goes, it's very straightforward, as low-carb dieting lends itself readily to being Reset. While there's no doubt that losing weight requires a reduction in calories, some low-carb diet plans cut calories far lower than would be liveable or enjoyable long term. Remember that if you're going to keep off the weight that you lose, you need to sustain whatever behaviors you've adopted to lose it in the first place.

The good news here is that low-carb diets confer a great deal of fullness or satiety all by themselves. Studies on non–calorie counting low-carb dieters reveal that eating very limited amounts of carbohydrates and high amounts of protein leads people to naturally consume nearly 500 fewer calories a day.[4] This might translate to a pound of loss weekly (and explain why these diets "work"). Furthermore, on low-carb diets, our bodies' natural carbohydrate storage unit, glycogen, is depleted, and as a result, in the first week or two there will be an additional 5- to 10-pound loss due to the water that's also lost. But don't kid yourself, those 5 to 10 pounds will return just as quickly as glycogen stores are built back up if you return to eating sufficient quantities of carbohydrates.

While some low-carb diet gurus are staunch opponents of tracking calories, for the life of me, I can't understand why. Studies on weight loss and dietary compositions have demonstrated that regardless of what you're eating, it's total calories that lead you to gain or lose. Calories are still the currency of weight; while I agree that low-carb diets naturally lead a person to consume fewer calories, even staunch low-carbers would find some caloric surprises if they explored their own foodscapes. Finding these surprises may also lead them to find easy swaps and adjustments that might help their overall weight management efforts. Don't forget, too, that as far as weight management behaviors go, none is more powerful than diarizing, perhaps even regardless of the numbers. The more frequently you consciously remind yourself of the changes you'd like to turn into habits, the more likely you'll actually do so. And the key to successful diarizing is entering into it nonjudgmentally and ensuring you use it to guide your decisions, not to make them.

If you'd like to try or to continue on a low-carb diet, follow the Reset principles as they're laid out here with low-carb as your backdrop. The main additions are to add in the food diary (though some low-carb dieters already track carbs) and ensure that you eat enough to be happily satisfied. Most people greatly enjoy carbohydrates; so while they may well have success with weight management going low-carb, the results will likely be temporary unless they can see themselves living the rest of their lives with markedly reduced amounts. At least 50 percent of my patients report that they easily lost more than 40 pounds on a low-carb diet at some point in their lives (according to a 2004 report on CNN, nearly one in five American households reported at least one member having been on a low-carb diet[5]), but that eventually, the carbohydrate restriction proved to be too traumatic for them to sustain; ultimately, they abandoned their strategies and regained their weight. So if you're interested in trying low-carb, by all means, go for it. But remember: you have to do it in a way that is not traumatic. You're not allowed to be hungry, or have cravings, or feel like your life isn't normal. If you're really keen on trying low-carb but feel unsatisfied, you might need to bring them back slowly and determine what amount of carbs you personally need in your life to be satisfied. There may still be benefit to fullness and satiety on lower, rather than truly low, carb approaches. And of course, I hope by now it goes without saying; if you're happy with a very low-carb life and feel you can live with it forever, please don't feel any medical pressure to quit.

CASE STUDY

Bob

Bob's a 49-year-old former jock who married his high school sweetheart, fathered three little girls, took on a desk job, and over time ended up tipping the scales at over 300 pounds. When we ran his blood work, he turned out to be markedly hyperinsulinemic. What that means is that in order to handle his body's blood sugar, his pancreas was pumping out nearly five times what I would consider to be a normal amount of insulin. Exploring Bob's past history with weight management revealed that he once lost 80 pounds over six months on the Atkins diet. Delving further,

he disclosed that the only reason he stopped was because his wife, a registered nurse, was worried that it was bad for his health. I asked that
he bring his wife with him to an appointment, and together we all discussed the facts around low-carb diets. Bob elected to go on a modified
low-carb diet, and in so doing, he gained some confidence as he knew it
had worked for him once before. The differences this time included more
regular meals and snacks, and tracking what he was consuming, which
allowed him to be a bit less strict than his first time around, "The first
time I did low-carb, I was scared a single piece of bread would sink me.
This time around, while I'm still careful, I realize that I don't need to be
perfect. Not needing to be perfect makes me much more confident that
I'll be able to stick to this approach for good."

RESETTING PALEO AND ANCESTRAL DIETS (PALEO SOLUTION, PRIMAL BLUEPRINT, PALEO ANSWER)

Boiled down to their common essence, paleo diets recommend we eat
like our Paleolithic ancestors did. The Paleolithic period began roughly
2.5 million years ago and ended roughly 10,000 years ago. These days,
paleo diets tend to consist of grass-fed meats, fish, seafood, vegetables
and root vegetables, fruits, and nuts. They usually shun grains, dairy, legumes, refined sugars, and oils (though some paleo folks are okay with
olive oil). At its most basic, if you can hunt it or gather it, it's usually good.

To date, there have been only a few small studies that have specifically
evaluated paleo diets for weight loss and/or health, but they have been
positive. For the record, I can't think of any reason why paleo diets would
be risky. I love paleo's emphasis on consuming whole, unadulterated, un-
processed foods, as doing so will almost certainly improve health, and
likely help with weight loss. Paleo diets usually necessitate actual cooking, which helps to get people away from both restaurants and reheatable,
hypercaloric, hyperprocessed boxed meals.

Resetting paleo diets couldn't be easier. They already place a great emphasis on protein, so including protein with every meal and snack will

be straightforward. Most paleo diets don't involve food diaries, so you'll need to add one, along with adding your promise not to undereat or over-restrict. If you try a paleo approach and you're painfully missing grains or dairy, bring back the smallest amount of dairy or grains that you need to feel you enjoy your dietary lifestyle enough to sustain it forevermore. Sure, you'll no longer be perfectly paleo, but as you must know by now, perfect's not really a worthwhile goal.

CASE STUDY

Emily

Dr. Emily Deans, a psychiatrist from Texas, had hit her highest weight. Her second pregnancy was coming to a close, and her scale was tipping 214 pounds—a long way away from the 130 pounds she weighed most of her pre-childbearing life. Looking back on her approaches to weight loss in the past, with her most successful effort coming through the popular but involved Body for Life program, she knew that given her far more hectic lifestyle today, what was workable pre-kids wouldn't be work-able now.

And it's not as if she had gained weight eating junk food. On the contrary, Dr. Deans had been following the advice of food writer and whole foods promoter Michael Pollan, and was cooking the vast majority of her meals from scratch. While certainly the pregnancy had a great deal to do with her gain, 10 months after giving birth she was frustrated that despite her healthy living, she hadn't lost all of her pregnancy weight.

It was then that she found paleo, and she's been living with it ever since. Her lifestyle is still as healthy as it gets. She home-cooks nearly everything, exercises vigorously for a minimum of three hours a week, and she never feels out of dietary control. But as she says about her paleo, "It's not pure, I cheat. Sometimes I'll have a slice of pizza, some dark choco-late, or a glass of wine."

Dr. Deans doesn't currently keep a food diary; she describes herself as a fairly routine eater, and her current foodscape without counting has led her to her pre-pregnancy weight. When I asked her what she would do differently if hypothetically she were living with her current lifestyle yet her weight wasn't where she felt it ought to be, she quickly answered, "I'd count more—I would figure out calories."

Dr. Deans is currently working on a paleo writing project with Mark Sisson. You can readily reach her both on Twitter (@evolutionarypsy) and on her own blog (evolutionarypsychiatry.blogspot.com).

RESETTING LOW-FAT DIETS (DASH DIET, FORKS OVER KNIVES, FUHRMAN, ORNISH, ESSELSTYN, EAT-CLEAN)

There are different sorts of low-fat diets, but likely their most popular rendition could be better described as plant-based low-fat diets. These have been shown to have real and tangible health benefits, especially for the prevention and/or management of heart disease. A fabulously inspirational documentary called *Forks over Knives* depicted a low-fat diet that places a tremendous emphasis on primarily plant-based from-scratch cooking. Unfortunately, that's not necessarily the low-fat diet adopted by the general public, who may rely on equally processed and boxed low-fat versions of higher fat, heavily processed foods. Therein lies the problem with low-fat diets. Governments the world over have recommended low-fat diets for the past 40 years or so; consequently, the food industry has responded by creating products that while certainly low in fat, are high in processed and refined carbohydrates. Basically, they took out fat but put in sugar, high-fructose corn syrup, and refined white flour. The thinking nowadays is that the rise in obesity and chronic disease in society may be in large part due to this phenomenon.

If you're going to adopt a low-fat approach, aim for one that puts an emphasis on cooking rather than relying on low-fat versions of your favorite processed staples. In resetting a low-fat diet, your primary challenge will be ensuring that there is protein in every meal and snack. Low-fat-friendly sources of protein include beans, soy-based products (tofu and its friends), lean meats, fish, seafood, low-fat dairy, and egg whites. If you're struggling to find low-fat snacks that are also high in protein, it may be worth experimenting with the three-meal-a-day option and forgoing the snacking. Aim for three higher-calorie meals, and try to ensure 25 percent of each meal's calories come from protein (otherwise you're simply going to end up hungry, and yes, I realize this is slightly higher than what Dr. Ornish recommends as an upper limit). The only other option would be to eat truly tremendous volumes of vegetables, beans, and other low-energy-dense foods, and while there's absolutely nothing wrong with doing so, it might be impractical for many; during a busy workday, finding the lengthy blocks of time required to eat large amounts of plant-based low-fat foods poses a logistical challenge.

CALCULATING THE PERCENTAGE OF YOUR DAY'S OR MEAL'S CALORIES COMING FROM PROTEIN

It's not difficult. You'll need to know total calories and total grams of protein. Once you've got both, it's just:

$$[(Protein\ grams) \times 4] \div Calories] \times 100$$

For those scared of formulas, simply take your protein grams, multiply by 4, divide by total calories—whatever comes after the decimal point is your protein percentage (e.g., 0.25 = 25 percent). ⊚

CASE STUDY

Tosca

Tosca Reno is a healthy living dynamo and almost a force of nature in the health and fitness world. She's the best-selling author of the Eat-Clean diet series, a motivational speaker, magazine columnist, wellness consultant, media personality, and 53-year-old swimsuit and fitness model. But she wasn't always all of those things. In fact, for much of her life she was unhappy, unfulfilled, overweight, and a serial traumatic dieter. She says, "From the ages of 17 to 39 I did all the usual things that people who don't know how to diet do—attempt to starve yourself or perform a great deal of exercise, but it was at 39 when I finally decided I had enough of that."

So what did Tosca do? At first she turned to fitness, but that took her only so far. It was when she began to explore the impact of eating "clean" that her puzzle pieces truly fell into place. She cut out processed foods from her life, began carefully reading food labels and ingredients lists, and focused on a diet consisting of lean proteins and complex carbohydrates.

Tosca's top weight was 204 pounds, but for the past 14 years she's stayed closer to the 135-pound mark. She credits her success to her style of eating. She's kept her weight steady for 14 years because the last diet she was ever on ended more than 14 years ago: "Eating clean works for me because it's a lifestyle way of managing your weight."

Tosca's healthy living approach is still an evolution. Tosca told me that over the course of the past few years she's made some changes to her choices, deemphasizing grains and increasing dietary fats from lean proteins and healthy fats to account for about 28 percent of her daily calories. While that style of eating can no longer be classified as low-fat, it shows you how real Tosca is, embracing change that works for her—the true hallmark of a person who's not on a diet.

For more information on Tosca and eating clean, you can pick up one of her many bestsellers, visit one of her popular websites, such as www .eatcleandiet.com and www.toscareno.com, or head to one of her many speaking appearances.

RESETTING VEGAN AND VEGETARIAN DIETS

I'll often get asked if vegan or vegetarian lifestyles are safe. The answer is most assuredly yes. As mentioned when I was talking about low-fat diets, plant-based eating has been regularly associated with decreased risks of chronic diseases, including heart disease—our number one killer. But there's one caveat with vegan diets: ensuring an adequate supply of what are often animal-based nutrients. Vitamin B_{12} is the nutrient most difficult to obtain from nonanimal sources, as it's simply not present in any useful amounts in plants. Consequently, strict vegans may be well advised to supplement with vitamin B_{12} as deficiencies, when severe, can cause a myriad of problems, some irreversible. Other nutrients that it may be worth asking your doctor to test for, if you're following a vegan diet, would include calcium, iron, vitamin D, selenium, phosphorous, and zinc.

I think the greatest challenge to resetting a vegan or vegetarian diet is ensuring the inclusion of protein with all meals and snacks. Soy-based products, lentils, beans, ancient grains, whole grains, and nuts work for vegans, and depending on the type of vegetarian you are, you may also have the option of eggs or dairy products.

As with resetting low-fat diets, if snacks with protein are challenging for you, consider the approach of three larger meals a day, ensuring that at least 25 percent of calories in each meal comes from protein.

CASE STUDY

Maryanne

I don't know if you remember Maryanne. She's the 39-year-old mother of two young girls who struggled with the guilt brought on by years of traumatic and overly restrictive dieting. Shortly after Maryanne enrolled in our program, her 12-year-old daughter decided to become a vegetarian. In part because she felt a dramatic change would do her good, Maryanne decided to follow along. This time, however, she decided that trying to become a "perfect" vegetarian would be a bad idea, and so she's become a home-based vegetarian—she'll still eat meat when she eats out in restaurants. The biggest change for Maryanne was learning new dishes, but six months later, she's doing great. "At first we were reliant on a great deal of pasta, but I found the calories were a real challenge to control. My advice to anyone trying to become a vegetarian is to make friends with lentils and tofu. They're much easier to cook with than they sound."

RESETTING WEIGHT WATCHERS, OVEREATERS ANONYMOUS, AND TOPS

I have my share of lifetime Weight Watchers members in my office's program. They've found me not because Weight Watchers is somehow inherently flawed, but rather because many people simply Weight Watch improperly.

The most common complaint I hear from lapsed Weight Watchers is that they were hungry on the plan. I wonder if that doesn't simply reflect the fact that it's a fairly common practice for Weight Watchers to save up the bulk of their day's points for dinner. I've also met many Weight Watchers who felt that their points were a ceiling and that when they went over, they felt tremendously guilty, or elected to eat crackers for dinner because they had no point room left for anything else. I've also met many Weight Watchers who found that their meetings focused almost entirely on absolute weight change as the be-all and end-all; in so doing, if a member didn't lose, they felt shamed or left out. Others reported that because at the end of the day it was all just about points, they felt they weren't eating healthfully and instead were just spending their points on small amounts of high-calorie junk food.

Generally speaking, Weight Watchers can be described as a low-fat diet that aims to provide a daily deficit of 1,000 calories. Their new Weight Watchers 360° program takes a slightly algorithmic approach to calorie allocations that is meant to take into account the differences in impact different types of food have on satisfaction and satiety. Like Reset, Weight Watchers has no forbidden foods and no required foods.

For some, a 1,000-calorie daily deficit will simply leave them hungry or craving. For all, saving calories for dinner will likely backfire with after-dinner cravings. And points? Unfortunately, there's a huge inter-product variation in calories. Slices of bread that are 50 percent higher in calories than other slices of bread may be scored by a Weight Watcher as equivalent in points. Same goes for muffins, bagels, pizza slices, and really anything that comes preportioned. Sure, you can actually plug in numbers to calculate points, but how many Weight Watchers honestly take the time to do so? And if they do, why not simply track calories in the first place? Weight Watchers 360° also gives fruit a freebie, yet if you have a large orange, a large apple, and a cup full of grapes a day, you'll be consuming more than a Snickers bar's worth of calories!

Resetting Weight Watchers isn't difficult, though. First, definitely don't save your points for dinner. Instead, divvy them up into quarters and have one-quarter of your points with each meal, and then divvy up the remaining quarter among three snacks. Don't forget to ensure that there's protein in every meal and snack. I also recommend you score fruit, as those calories can easily add up. Easiest way there: 2 points for a large, 1 point for a small. (I'd be willing to wager that when the next point system is unveiled, fruit will once again be scored.) If you go over your points total, don't sweat it. Your goal is the smallest number of points that you need to be satisfied, not some prescribed total you're never allowed to exceed. Lastly, don't let folks in meetings make you feel badly about your efforts. The scale measures what you weigh, not how you're doing, and if you live and die by the scale, you'll probably die by the scale because some weeks you're simply going to weigh more than you feel you should based on how you're doing.

Of course, I'd prefer it if instead of points, you tracked calories. Log onto this book's website at TheDietFix.com and calculate your caloric needs, and Reset along with the group support you receive from your local Weight Watchers chapter.

As far as Resetting Overeaters Anonymous or TOPS, that's as simple as following Reset principles and heading over to OA or TOPS meetings for support. Given the benefits seen in studies looking at weight loss buddies, that may be a wise plan for those who may not feel comfortable sharing their journey with their friends or families.

RESETTING A MEAL REPLACEMENT PROGRAM (OPTIFAST, HMR, ISAGENIX, IDEAL PROTEIN)

This one's a toughie. Are you really going to live a life with meal replacements forever? Where these programs shine in clinical practice is when they're used as pre–weight loss surgery diets with the aim of helping a person rapidly lose weight immediately prior to surgery—and in so doing cause their livers to shrink, allowing for better surgical access and decreased surgical risk.

If you're going to go on one of these diets to kick-start your weight loss and plan to Reset down the road, of course you can do so and use Reset to try to ease yourself back into the real eating world. But my recommendation would instead just be to Reset from the get-go; while you'll absolutely lose weight more slowly, you'll be that much more likely to keep the weight you lose off.

The reason I'm not fond of the kick-started approach to weight management is that in a sense, it's twice as difficult. The difficulty in lifestyle change is change itself. You'll need to change the way you're living during your kick-start, and then you'll need to change the way you're living again to try to keep off the weight you've lost. But if change itself is the challenge, by adopting a lose-weight one way, keep-it-off another way approach, you're just giving yourself twice as many opportunities to struggle, since you're giving yourself twice as many changes to undertake. If you give yourself twice as many opportunities to struggle, you might be twice as likely to get frustrated—and get frustrated often enough and you might just give up on change altogether.

The other option is a mixed use of these diets. For instance, many people don't enjoy or don't have time for breakfast. Using a high-protein meal replacement for breakfast may be something those folks could do happily for life. Meal replacements may also be useful products and plans in a pinch if the option is skipping the meal altogether versus quickly downing a meal replacement shake; shake wins over skipping. In fact, most mornings I drink a protein shake, and while it's homemade (the recipe's included in this book), the principle's the same. Though I have to say, when I eat my breakfast rather than drink it, my fullness factor is somewhat heightened.

RESETTING AN INTERMITTENT FASTING PROGRAM (THE 8-HOUR DIET, EAT. STOP. EAT, LEANGAINS, THE FAST DIET, THE 5:2 DIET)

You might think that intermittent fasting (IF) wouldn't lend itself to being Reset as by definition IF will involve very lengthy periods of time between meals and snacks. However, given the primary principle of being Reset is actually enjoying your life enough to keep living with it, certainly if you were happily satisfied with an IF-style approach, I wouldn't want you to try to live otherwise. Broadly, there are three common IF approaches: Martin Berkhans' Leangains (repackaged last year into the bestselling *8-Hour Diet*), which includes a daily 8-hour window within which eating is permitted, followed by 16 hours of fasting, Brad Pilon's Eat. Stop. Eat, which involves once or twice weekly 24-hour fasts followed by thoughtful eating, and Krista Varady's, which involves eating 500 to 600 calories total for two days each week.

Resetting these programs is straightforward and would involve the inclusion of a food diary, ensuring there's protein with every meal or snack, regular cooking, and the honest evaluation of a dietary style that in turn might lead to more suffering than is permanently enjoyable. Consequently, if while trying IF you find hunger to be a regular fight, IF might not be the right approach for you. Anecdotally, I've been told that with each approach, the struggle with hunger dissipates over the course of the first two to four weeks of practice, so if you do consider adopting one of these styles of eating, you might want to see if a few weeks of toughing it out doesn't lead to an easier, and for some, a permanently enjoyable lifestyle.

CASE STUDY

Dick

"I was a really fat kid," is how Dick Talens, now a New York City fitness guru and cofounder of Fitocracy, the social network fitness app, described himself before he found intermittent fasting. Dick's story isn't all that uncommon. Overweight childhood, lots of screen time, and too many calories. But his is a success story, albeit one of multiple stages.

When Dick first wanted to lose weight, he started with the brute force method. "I ate a ham sandwich and a bowl of soup per day. I lost 60 to 70 pounds, but I was absolutely miserable." Soon thereafter, he channeled his brute-forced dietary efforts into actual brute force and fell in love with bodybuilding. Between the ages of 17 and 22, he started eating more regularly. The pattern he started out with is the one I tend to start everyone off with: he was eating five to six smaller meals and snacks spread out throughout the day. While he did well with his weight and fitness, he still struggled around food. According to Dick, he missed eating large amounts in single meals, and mealtime would often leave him feeling "underwhelmed." Then Dick found intermittent fasting (IF).

While some forms of IF include 24-hour fasts one to two times per week, Dick follows the Leangains advice of IF guru and Swedish personal trainer Martin Berkhan, which gives him eight-hour daily windows during which eating is permitted. Dick organized his life around a large meal at 1:00 p.m., followed by another large meal at 9:00 p.m. (many other IF'ers will have three meals during that eight-hour window). At first, he reports, "I had a lot of trouble starting with intermittent fasting," but soon thereafter he describes how for the first time in his life he felt "not enslaved by food."

There's theoretical and even experimental science that backs up intermittent fasting as a healthy option. The only thing that really matters is that IF has allowed Dick to control his calories, repair his relationship with food, and enjoy his life—the very foundation of being Reset.

RESETTING A DIET NOT LISTED HERE

Reset can be boiled down into one exceedingly simple principle and cardinal rule: you need to enjoy your life even as you are changing the way you live it. If you don't like it, you won't stick to it. Full stop.

There are thousands of different diets out there. Each and every one of them works so long as you consume fewer calories than you're burning. And if you enjoy the life you're living while following any approach, who am I to suggest you should change?

To Reset any program, the main must-have is a food diary. With it, you'll be able to track not only the calories you're consuming, but also the sustainability of the diet, since by tracking your day's degree of difficulty you'll be able to tell whether you're enjoying your life. If you're struggling with hunger or cravings, you'll need to add more calories. Try to ensure that protein's well distributed and that you're adding low-energy-density foods to pump up your dietary volume, but if after that's all said and done your days are still difficult, it may mean it's time for you to consider another approach.

Clearly, if weight or health is one of your primary priorities or concerns, you're going to need to make some real dietary compromises. My prescription for chocolate is not all-you-can-eat. Instead it's a "the-smallest-amount-you-need-to-be-satisfied" one, which of course will be determined in part by your own personal health and weight priorities.

LIVE

Now that you've realized that you can Reset most every diet program, there are some hurdles and issues that you will undoubtedly face from time to time living a real life. From travel, to medications, to scales, and a great deal in between, let's delve deeper into the behaviors and attitudes you'll want to cultivate to help put an end to your days of traumatic dieting.

VACATION STRATEGIES

Though I haven't seen the studies to prove it, I've heard that the average weight gain during a week of cruising nears seven pounds, and I've certainly seen plenty of folks gain four to five pounds during a weeklong stay at an all-inclusive resort. Once you factor in alcohol, buffets, and disorganized eating, you can start to understand how this could happen. But let me give you a little more detail about what this means. Those are some hefty numbers, as to gain one pound a week you need to eat *at least* 3,500 more calories than you burn. Most folks, especially folks who have weight to lose, are likely burning between 1,800 and 2,800 calories daily; so to gain those kinds of numbers they need to be consuming in the neighborhood of 6,000 calories a day at a minimum.

That's the caloric equivalent of eating a McDonald's Quarter Pounder every waking hour from eight in the morning until eleven o'clock at night.

So how do you get by?

My Top 10 List of Vacation Strategies

1. Eat every two and a half to three and a half hours and make sure to have breakfast within 30 to 60 minutes of waking up. Not eating frequently and leaving too long between meals and snacks can lead to evening hunger. Hunger plus alcohol plus vacationing plus a buffet leads to—in the case of cruising—literally boatloads of calories.

2. Control breakfast. Try to minimize breakfast buffets and/or the classic bacon, egg, toast, and home fries. Having those will likely lead you to consume 650 to 1,000 calories before your morning snack and certainly makes it tougher to keep calories reasonably managed. A safe eating out breakfast for vacations would be some very gently buttered (or dry) whole grain toast to dip into some freshly poached eggs, along with a side of some cottage cheese, yogurt, and/or fresh fruit—still an indulgent breakfast, but less than half the calories of the classic American breakfast of two eggs, two pieces of toast, bacon, sausage, and home fries.

3. Eat your fruit, don't drink it. Or at least don't drink it regularly. Yes, freshly squeezed juices are a wonderful indulgence, but figure that the tall glass of orange juice you just downed had the calorie equivalent of more than three oranges and drop for drop the same amount of calories and sugar as Coca-Cola (which I hope goes without saying should be avoided). That giant piña colada or other fruity alcohol concoction? If it's like those I've had at resorts, each one's packing a Big Mac's worth of calories.

4. Include protein with every meal and snack. Snack-wise, 30 almonds have just over 200 calories and nearly 8 grams of protein. Most important, they won't melt down by the pool, will go well with an ice-cold beverage, and can be purchased nearly everywhere, and if they're not around, I'd guarantee that peanuts are.

5. Try the à la carte restaurants rather than the buffets. Most resorts will have both buffets and à la carte restaurants. À la carte, you're less likely to be tempted to really load up; just as important, the food's usually better so you'll actually enjoy what you're eating more. You might even consider booking your dinner reservations a few weeks before your trip, as often the à la carte restaurants have limited seating and fill up fast. If you do happen to hit the buffet, consider using the smaller salad plate to trick your brain into being satisfied with a smaller portion.

6. Booze after the meal. Alcohol is an appetite stimulant and affects your ability to make decisions thoughtfully. It also dissolves resolve. If you are a drinker, if you can hold off on the drinking until after you've eaten, you're less likely to overdo it.

7. Be prepared. While you may need to rely on restaurants for your meals, certainly you can pack your own snacks or buy them wherever you are. As noted previously, prepackaged nuts are available from hotel gift stores and don't melt by the pool, and protein bars can be found in almost any drugstore or supermarket, at least in North America.

8. Use your mini-bar to store fruits, cheeses, and yogurts. Most hotels will be happy to empty your mini-bar before you arrive if you call ahead to request it. Not only will it remove the temptation of overpriced snacks, it will also give you a place where you can store some actual groceries. You can buy fruits, cheeses, yogurt, and so on (or pilfer them from the buffet; if it's all inclusive, you've already paid for it!) and have them all on hand for easy snacking or an in-room breakfast. Even if your hotel doesn't have a mini-bar in every room, it's worth calling the front desk and asking if they have mini-fridges—many do as some guests will be traveling with medications that require refrigeration. Some hotels will also have mini-microwaves available for those who ask.

9. Grilled seafood is your friend, as is sashimi. Seafood's naturally low in calories and high in protein, and given that many vacations are seaside, it'll be fresh and delicious to boot. A quick word of seafood caution, though— sushi can often be quite high in calories. It may be worth exploring the calorie content in your favorite sushi pieces with an online database (such as www.calorieking.com) to enable more informed choices, though sashimi (raw fish) is always a reliably lower calorie choice.

10. Don't slap your wrist too hard. It's better to indulge thoughtfully and gain a pound or two than to be excessively strict and have you one step closer to abandoning your excessively strict weight management effort altogether.

I'd also encourage you to continue to keep your food diary on the road, but don't feel the need to be even remotely accurate with calories. Of course, if calorie counts are available for the restaurants you frequent it's worth using them, but if not, I'd prefer you simply entered in guesstimates than stop your records altogether. By keeping your food diary on vacation, even if wildly inaccurate, it will keep the act of diarizing itself alive, whereas if you quit, it may be difficult to start up again on your return. Given that you'll just be guessing, record keeping on the road should take no more than a minute a day, and doing so will also serve to consciously remind you to remain thoughtful.

BUSINESS TRIPS AND CONFERENCES

For business trips and conferences, many of the same tips apply, and here are a few more.

1. If you can, and especially if the business trip is lengthy, try to book yourself into a suite-style hotel that has a kitchen or kitchenette in your room. While I certainly wouldn't suggest you cook all of your meals, taking control of some of them will help you maintain far greater control over your calories. Consider having breakfast in your room, and for every week you're gone, aim for at least two homemade dinners.

2. If you happen to go to the same locations over and over again, especially if they're large cities, and you're in a suite-style hotel, consider

employing a local food delivery service to have some staples ready and waiting for you in your fridge upon arrival. You might also want to look into whether or not that city has a calorie-controlled meal-delivery service available, as these are definitely growing in popularity.

3. For conferences where large buffets are the norm, resist the urge of getting in line first, and instead hang back. Chances are by the time you get to the front of the line, some of the most indulgent choices will be gone, reducing the temptation to you. You'll also have time to scope out what's being offered to allow you to better plan what you'd like to eat. Remember, too, that even at the conferences I go to, the ones with doctors involved in the research or clinical management of obesity, the snacks are awful—huge calorific muffins, might-as-well-be-chocolate-bar granola bars, and sugary soft drinks. Don't forget to pack or buy your own snacks.

WEEKENDS!

Does this sound like you: lose weight Monday through Friday and gain it back on the weekend?

It's one of the many unfairnesses of weight management: two quick days can easily erase a week of best intentions.

How does that happen?

Weekends are actually pretty long—a full 28.57 percent of your week. I know it doesn't feel that way but, indeed, weekends take up almost a third of our lives. Get disorganized, go out to eat a few times, have a few drinks or simply have a "write-off," and suddenly nearly a third of your week is lost. For folks actively trying to lose weight, a weekend of even minor indulgences can easily erase two to three days of great efforts, leaving a person with just a day or two a week to lose. Have life throw a hiccup or two on those days, or have a real blowout, and you can kiss your week's weight loss good-bye even if the majority of the week you were actually doing great. Five steps forward and two steps back when it comes to weekends often translates to five steps forward and five steps back.

To put some numbers to this, let's say during the workweek, through your own personal strategies (be they balanced deficits, low-carb, counting points, exercise, combination approaches), you managed to create a true 400-calorie daily deficit. Enjoyed daily, that would likely lead you to lose a pound every 8 to 12 days, allowing for some differences in individual variation in energy efficiencies.

But then the weekend comes. You might go out with friends (food is an essential part of our celebratory and social lives); you might be less organized about eating and invite more of a hormonal drive to eat; you might want to kick back and have a few drinks to unwind. Truthfully, given the calorific world we live in, it wouldn't be difficult at all to amass 800-calorie daily surpluses over the weekend, rather than 400-calorie deficits.

Then it's back to your workweek, and even if you're fabulous about getting right back to calorie deficit–inducing behaviors, you'll be spending Monday through Thursday just erasing your weekend surpluses, leaving you with only one lonely day a week to actually lose weight.

I don't preach that weekends can't be indulgent. I don't tell people to stop eating out. And I don't tell people they're not allowed to drink. We're on this planet once, and for many, indulgences on weekends are a welcome end to the workweek. However, I do preach that at the very least, you should ensure that your weekends are well organized in terms of food, so that if you do indulge, you are choosing to do so because it's worth it and not just needlessly undoing all of the great progress you've made the other five days of the week because you got hungry.

Weekends need to follow the same rules as the week. Eat every two and a half to three and a half hours, be calorie aware, and eat out only for celebration. Don't waste your calories eating in a food court because you didn't plan your day's shopping well, or lounge around until 11:00 a.m. only to have a 2,000-calorie brunch just because it's Sunday.

If you're serious about weight management, your efforts need to occur seven days of the week. Those efforts need to include minimizing hunger with well-organized meals, snacks, and macronutrients, and knowing what you're eating. It doesn't mean don't indulge; it just means ensure that hunger doesn't fuel your indulgences and instead you've consciously thought about them and have decided they're actually worth their calories to you.

For many, weekends unravel not because they're filled with revelry, but rather because they tend toward being less organized. There's no daily routine like there is during a workweek, and consequently there are fewer time-orienting cues that might help to remind you to eat. To fight this I recommend devising your own planning system, in which at the start of each weekend day you take just a few moments to think up your "food plan." It may be as simple as setting a recurrent Saturday and Sunday morning reminder on your smartphone or computer asking you "Do you have a food plan?," which once noticed will allow you to map out your day and may lead you to pack snacks, research the calories in restaurants you may be frequenting, and set alarms to remind you when it's time to eat.

HOLIDAYS

For many who battle with weight, holidays can be times of stress; more often than not, folks adopt one of two equally detrimental but diametrically opposite coping strategies—I'll call them the wrist-slappers and the write-offers.

The wrist-slappers are traumatic dieters who believe that long-term success with their weight depends solely on "willpower," on being able to "resist temptation," to "just push away from the table," or to simply avoid placing themselves in situations where high-calorie options are available. These are often hard-core dieters who on an annual or semiannual basis decide to "buckle down" and lose the weight, and then inevitably gain it back when they get sick of suffering.

The write-offers are the folks who are concerned about their weight but figure because it's a holiday they needn't think about calories at all. They'll eat what they want, when they want, with their only consideration as to amount being pleasure. These are often folks who believe in "cheat days" and who regularly make excuses for why they needn't think about the foods they're consuming. Birthdays, office parties, religious holidays, vacations, and even highly stressful days become write-offs. Then the write-offs spill over to days that they've "blown it," weekends, and busy times at work. These folks can easily gain three to five pounds a week during their days of abandon.

Instead of wrist-slaps and write-offs, how about thoughtfulness? That's where the only limits are imposed thoughtfully. You take stock of the situation, factor in the date or circumstance, and then consider the calories of any indulgence by asking yourself those two questions, *Is it worth the calories?* and *How much of that do I need to be happy?*

I figure everyone's got a food that fits into a line like:

"A Christmas without ___ for dinner/dessert just wouldn't be Christmas."

Make sure you fill in your blank thoughtfully, and really think about how much of that food is going to be a satisfying amount, and then savor and enjoy it without feeling guilt that you indulged, or bitterness that you abstained.

NEW YEAR'S RESOLUTIONS

These deserve a special mention as many people who think they're making resolutions *aren't*; instead, they're setting themselves up with goals or hopes, while resolutions are plans.

A goal might be to lose weight; to get in shape; to eat healthier; to love better; and to get a promotion.

A resolution is a plan that might actually get you to your goal. If, for instance, weight loss is your goal, then your resolutions may be to pack your lunches every day for work; to keep a food diary; and to put an end to all convenience meals out.

And of course, resolutions don't need New Year's to be initiated. Why not figure out some goals right now, and then craft their corresponding resolutions?

The Worst Weight-Related Resolutions

The first is resolving to simply "eat less."

How are you going to do that? Are you simply going to take smaller portions? Are you going to "cut back"?

That's your plan?

If it were that easy, do you think weight would be anyone's concern?

If all it took to lose weight was for people to simply "eat less," the world would be skinny.

Remember, what we choose to put on our plates reflects a sort of personal homeostasis—that we put as much food on our plates as we feel we need to be satisfied, and those needs include physiological needs, psychological needs, and even hedonistic needs. So what happens if you try to simply "cut back" without actually making any formative changes to the foods you eat or your timing of meals and snacks is that you end up dissatisfied. If all you're doing is plating the same food, following the same eating patterns as before, but just plating less, at least one of those needs will be left unmet. As a consequence you'll wind up feeling hungry, shortchanged, or bitter, and chances are your overly simplified resolution isn't going to make it past February.

You need to actually like your life with fewer calories. In order to do that, you're going to need to reformat your dietary organization so that you're using food in a manner that leads to less hunger and consequently more control—and in so doing, actually need less to be satisfied.

And it's not just about liking your life, it's also about liking your solution, and that brings me to the second worst weight-related resolution—extremes.

What do I mean?

Too many people make far too dramatic, broad, general, or strict resolutions and are then surprised when they quickly lose steam.

It's this phenomenon that pays the bills at every gym in the world—people take a flying leap into an overly aggressive and/or time-intensive program and, surprise, when they get sick of trying to bite off more than they can chew, they stop biting.

The thing about flying leaps? You tend to land on your face, whereas if you take small steps, you may actually get somewhere.

Even if you enjoy healthy eating and exercise, overdoing them isn't a wise plan. Reality television teaches you to try to lose huge amounts of weight each and every week; to restrict, deny, and avoid dietary indulgences; that exercise, in order to be useful, needs to be performed in massive amounts (often to the point of throwing up) and be painful.

And while those strategies may well work for contestants on a reality television show, they sure aren't going to work well for a working mom with three kids on three different sports teams, or in my case, a working dad with three kids and a blog, who's also writing a book.

The more weight you want to permanently lose, the more of your lifestyle you're going to have to permanently change. Trying to adopt changes you don't like is a surefire way to ensure that they're not going to be permanent.

So this year, resolve to like your resolutions. Analyze each and every one by asking *Can I happily keep living this way?* Do you really think that you'll be able to wake up to exercise at 5:30 every morning? Are you really never going to have alcohol, chocolate, or chips again? Take your time and, using the principles discussed during Reset's goal-setting Day 9, build some resolutions you can be happy with. Because if you can't do it happily, you're probably not going to keep doing it.

EAT

During your Reset, you made friends with food, and we also just discussed some strategies for specific occasions like vacations and business meetings. We've talked about different styles of diets and the importance of different macronutrients. But there's a great deal more to dietary behavior than simply the venue or your diet's composition. After all, food's not just fuel.

If it were, we'd have calorie tablets and everyone would probably be pretty darn skinny.

Food's a lot of different things to a lot of different people, but for all of us at different times, food is friendship, comfort, solace, celebration, and cheer.

And food pretty much never lets you down.

You could have the best marriage, kids, parents, job, hobby, friends in the world, but from time to time, with each of those, you'll hit some rough patches.

Your comfort food, on the other hand? It's a constant. Whenever you need it and whatever you need it for, it'll deliver. Each and every time.

Food's power isn't only something that shouldn't be overlooked; rather, it is something that should be exploited. The key consideration here, though, is ensuring that when you do choose to allow food to play a role of comfort and celebration, you do so thoughtfully, and that "it's worth it." I want to take you through some considerations to that question that you may not have heard about.

PERHAPS A CALORIE'S NOT A CALORIE

File this one under cool data!

A simple study published in *Food and Nutrition Research*[1] looked at the differences between whole foods and processed foods, specifically at the calories the body utilizes to metabolize them (something called "diet induced thermogenesis," also known as the thermic effect of food). Absorbing nutrients and digesting the foods we consume burns calories itself, and the researchers wondered whether heavily processed foods required fewer calories to digest than their whole food alternatives. Eighteen subjects were enrolled in a crossover study (meaning they all ate both test and control meals), and the thermic effect of food was measured following the ingestion of two different cheese sandwiches.

One cheese sandwich was made with cheddar cheese and a multi-grain bread containing whole sunflower seeds and whole grains, while the other sandwich was made with white bread and processed cheese. Both sandwiches contained the same number of calories.

The results?

While subjects reported that the whole food sandwich was tastier, both sandwiches conferred equal levels of satiety. But eating the whole food sandwich led to roughly double the thermic effect of food as the processed sandwich, an effect that lasted nearly an hour longer than that of the processed meal.

Why wasn't this surprising?

Whole grains take longer to digest due to the protective fibrous sheath that processing removes. We also would expect the whole grain sandwich to have more protein and fat (which it did), which in turn delays the speed with which the body is able to break down the accompanying carbohydrates.

So what does all of this mean to someone who is interested in calories?

It means it takes more energy to release the nutrients of the whole food sandwich, with the differences between the meals resulting in a 9.7 percent increase in the net energy gain of the processed food meal. In other words: eat processed crap and you're effectively burning 10 percent *fewer* calories per meal than you would be were you eating healthier whole food alternatives with the equivalent number of calories.

Now, this was a small study, and it's too soon to extrapolate from this across the board, but were it to be true for all processed foods—given their viral spread across the developed world these past 30 years, and given that a 10 percent net energy gain is huge—this might be another great reason to ditch the Wonder Bread and Velveeta.

ARE ARTIFICIAL SWEETENERS SAFE?

Of all the manmade food additives, perhaps none is more vilified than artificial sweeteners, and yet they're likely the most studied food additives in history.

Take aspartame, for instance. No doubt it receives the lion's share of fear out there. To date, aspartame has been deemed safe for human consumption by the independent regulatory agencies of more than 90 countries worldwide. A massive meta analysis of the literature on aspartame concluded:

> The studies provide no evidence to support an association between aspartame and cancer in any tissue. The weight of existing evidence is that aspartame is safe at current levels of consumption as a nonnutritive sweetener.[2]

while the European Union's own massive aspartame review concluded:

> The Committee concluded that on the basis of its review of all the data in animals and humans available to date, there is no evidence to suggest that there is a need to revise the outcome of the earlier risk assessment or the ADI previously established for aspartame.[3]

There have also been grumblings about how artificial sweeteners increase appetite, challenge weight loss, and lead to various other unsavory outcomes. Yet when examining those studies, we see they're often exceedingly poorly designed, or are looking at all comers without controlling properly for dietary choices. Take, for instance, the study that made headlines in the winter of 2012, that said artificial sweeteners increase the risk of strokes.[4] That study shouldn't have ever been published. The authors didn't even attempt to control for dietary quality. What does that mean? As I'm sure you're aware, what we eat has a tremendous impact upon our risk of developing various chronic diseases. Consequently, not accounting for the folks who ate 10 meals a week from fast food restaurants, take-out places, or diners, versus those who actually ate at home and transformed raw ingredients, would likely skew the data. Worse still, if all you actually analyzed was amounts of consumed protein, carbohydrates, and fats, you'd fail miserably at usefully comparing the quality and caliber of the diets you were studying. By not looking at the quality of the diets, you'd be comparing quinoa to white rice, salmon to bacon, olive oil to Crisco. Yet that's exactly what the authors did. And it's not at all implausible that folks who regularly indulge in lower-caliber dietary choices assuage some of their dietary guilt and build their own health halos by choosing a diet beverage over a fully loaded one when consuming a less than healthful meal.

When you look at studies of folks who are either trying to lose weight or maintain a weight loss, not surprisingly the use of artificial sweeteners has been shown to be beneficial. One study looking at the National Weight Control Registry's Weight Loss Masters (in this case, folks who'd maintained at least a 10 percent weight loss for 11.5 years) found that the Masters consumed three times more servings daily of artificially sweetened soft drinks than the general population.[5] Another study that looked at the use of aspartame incorporated into the weight loss phase of a weight management program showed that study subjects assigned to the aspartame-sweetened group lost and kept off nearly 50 percent more weight than subjects assigned to abstain from artificially sweetened products.[6]

While data on aspartame do in fact suggest it's both safe and useful in weight management, the same cannot be said to be true about sugar. So do I recommend artificially sweetened beverages?

Yes and no.

In an ideal world, we'd drink far fewer sweet beverages. Whether our beverages are sweetened by means of sugar or by means of artificial sweeteners, having palates craving cloyingly sweet isn't going to help us in navigating through lower calorie choices or healthy fare. For many, liquid calories are the low-hanging fruit of weight management—easy to reduce. Consequently, I think it's certainly worth your own personal exploration of liquid calories. If indeed you're drinking huge amounts of them, especially sugar-sweetened ones, and you think you can use artificially sweetened beverages as a step-down strategy as you reduce the sweet drinks overall, I say go for it.

As far as I'm concerned, everyone's end goal is simply the smallest number of liquid calories they need to be satisfied and, ideally, the smallest amount of "sweet" beverages regardless of how the beverages got their "sweet" in the first place.

ALCOHOL

Yes, there are a great many calories in alcohol. Gram per gram, alcohol has more calories than carbohydrates or proteins and only slightly fewer than fats, but you might never know it because alcohol is exempt from listing its calories on nutrition labels. As a consequence, many folks are completely unaware of alcohol's caloric punch. How big a punch? Compared with Coca-Cola, per drop, wine has more than double the calories.

Certainly controlling alcohol is important, and while alcohol in moderation has been shown to be heart healthy, the same body of research looking at the health benefits of alcohol didn't control for weight. That means it's entirely possible that the health benefits of alcohol consumption may be outweighed by its weight and caloric contribution.

For folks who are capable of consuming alcohol in moderation, it's about the smallest amount you need to enjoy your life. For folks who are all or nothing, I recommend erring on the side of nothing.

To try to reduce alcohol consumption without having to think about it much, I've got a few suggestions for you to consider.

Smaller Glasses

Brains are strange places. Four ounces of wine just barely filling the bottom of a giant goblet will be far less satisfying psychologically than four ounces of wine completely filling an elegant four-ounce glass. Buying some rich-feeling, smaller glasses may be an easy way to trick your brain into enjoying less wine.

Spritzers

If you must go with the larger glasses, consider making spritzers by adding soda water to smaller quantities of wine, and in so doing again satisfying the primitive brain that is looking for a full glass.

Buy Better Booze

Let's say you spend $60 weekly on wine, splitting four $15 bottles with your spouse or partner. Why not instead buy, enjoy, and savor one $60 bottle weekly? You'll certainly be less likely to drink it mindlessly; you'll also have the added bonus of being able to explore the rich world of fine wines. To stretch the wine further, consider investing in an argon-canister wine preserver (available in any fine wine shop); after each time you drink, argon gas is inserted into the bottle, displacing the oxygen and preserving the wine, to allow you to sip it carefully all week long while perfectly preserving its flavor and character.

Mock-ohol

Sometimes drinking is more about peer pressure than it is about actually wanting a drink. Whether it's with clients or with pushy friends, not matching them drink for drink may be seen as a professional or personal slight. In those cases, consider ordering drinks that look like they're alcoholic. Tonic water alone can pass for a gin and tonic, diet ginger ale with no ice for beer, and so on. You can keep your hands busy and appear like you're keeping up without having to load up on the calories.

Your Best-Bet Booze

Of the drinks you enjoy, which has the fewest calories? Figuring that out will, at the very least, allow you to reduce your alcohol calories some.

For example, if your general pattern was two coolers a night, by switching to light beer or to sipping whisky you could still have two drinks a night, but you'd cut your alcohol calories by nearly 60 percent:

1½-oz jigger rye/scotch/bourbon/vodka = 103 calories
12-oz bottle light beer   = 103 calories
5-oz glass wine   = 125 calories
6-oz plain martini   = 135 calories
12-oz bottle regular beer   = 150 calories
6-oz screwdriver   = 180 calories
16-oz draft beer   = 203 calories
6-oz Cosmopolitan   = 213 calories
6-oz apple martini   = 235 calories
6-oz flavored cooler   = 240 calories
6-oz Long Island Iced Tea   = 276 calories

ARE YOUR PORTIONS AUTOMATED?

What's portion paralysis?

That's when your brain and your eyes have become so accustomed to a particular portion size for a particular meal that sticking with it is wholly automatic.

But sometimes it's wise to reduce portions.

Take me, for instance. In December 2010, I injured my back—pretty badly, in fact. My exercise regime went out the window. Rehab was very slow. Despite knowing better, I didn't adjust my portions with my drop-off in exercise and sure enough, over three months' time, I gained some weight. When I realized what was going on, I resumed keeping a careful food diary and recognized which were my higher-calorie meals.

One simple meal really struck me. It was pita pizza—a go-to meal for when I'm in a hurry and I want comfort-y food. It's not terrifically low in calories—each pita pizza has anywhere between 300 and 450 calories, depending on what I put on it. For most of my adult life, I'd have made three pitas' worth, and so my simple quick fix, when seeing such a high number, was to downshift my pita pizza portion to have only two. But when I was in a hurry or distracted, despite mentally deciding to eat less, sometimes I'd just forget and three would mindlessly appear in front of me.

It's not that two isn't satisfying, It's just that after years of always having three, I automatically revert to my established larger portions unless I consciously challenge my portion sizes.

My experience with the pita pizzas has led me to consciously challenge all of my automated portions prior to cooking or plating, and more often than not, I'm having just a tiny bit less than what had become habitual. More important, I'm not missing what's gone. On those rare circumstances when I'm not fully satisfied, either I'll go back for a thoughtful more or perhaps I'll have an after-dinner snack, but to be honest, it happens very infrequently.

A BIT MORE INCENTIVE TO EAT YOUR VEGETABLES

We all know that vegetables are good for us, but that doesn't always lead us to decide to eat them. If you're looking for another good reason to eat your vegetables, consider this: if you hide them in your food, you may need fewer calories to get full.

A recent study[7] out of Dr. Barbara Rolls' Volumetrics lab found that incorporating pureed vegetables into three- to five-year-olds' bread, pasta sauce, and chicken noodle casseroles reduced their energy intakes by an average of 12 percent! For five-year-olds, 12 percent amounted to 142 calories less a day, but there's no reason to think that this effect would be seen only in children; Dr. Rolls has shown these same types of effects over and over again in adults. Consequently, if you're aiming for 1,600 calories a day but you're finding yourself closer to 1,800, playing "hide the vegetables" may help you get those calories down.

Why does it happen? Decreasing the energy density of food (the calories per gram of the food you're eating) by adding piles of low-in-calories vegetables into your meals means if you eat the same portion you always eat, you'll consume fewer calories overall.

ARE YOU STUCK IN A DIETARY PIGEONHOLE?

I've said it before and I'll say it again: life is not about being perfect. But for too many people, it's all or nothing; they force themselves to comply to a rigid regime, and beat themselves up (or quit entirely!) at the first deviation. Striving to be perfect is a sure way to fall off the wagon.

Dietary pigeonholes often beg for perfection. Declare yourself a staunch anything, food-wise (low-carb, paleo, vegan, low-fat), and suddenly you'll have that many more opportunities to let yourself down. And if you let yourself down often enough, you're liable to quit whatever strategy it is that keeps making you feel guilty.

Sure, if you want to advocate a particular style of eating, go for it, just don't beat yourself up if you're not perfectly adherent.

Don't strive for perfection, and don't live in a pigeonhole. Instead do and eat your best, and rather than worry if your best isn't perfect, worry if it is.

DISENGAGE YOUR INDULGENCE AUTOPILOT!

It's something I hear about frequently when I meet new patients:

> *"Friday is pizza night."*
> *"Every Thursday, the gang at work goes out for dim sum at lunch."*
> *"After the kids' game on Saturday mornings, we do drive-thru Tim Horton's and share 20 Timbits."*

Now, I'm not knocking any of those choices directly. While certainly they're not *healthy* choices, and while I might even label them as nutritionally "bad" foods, the fact is they might be great indulgent choices.

What I mean to say is whether it's pizza, Chinese food, or doughnuts, if those are part of your life's seminal guilty dietary indulgences, then I think you probably owe it to yourself to continue to have them. Blindly restricting them now will likely lead you to totally abandon whatever overly strict healthy living strategy you've adopted later.

That said, you might want to take a moment to ask yourself a question like *Is the fact that it's Friday a good enough reason to order in pizza?*

Ultimately, when it comes to dietary indulgences and hedonistic pleasure, the question isn't, *Are you allowed?* Rather it's, *Is it worth it?* and *How much do I need to be satisfied?* Sometimes the answers may be *No* and *None* and other times significantly more than that. As mentioned earlier, I'm thinking you'll be eating far more indulgent foods on *your* birthday than you'll be eating on *my* birthday. But just because it's Friday? I'm guessing you can do better.

Disengage your indulgence autopilot and thoughtfully navigate your nutritional skies!

ARE YOU SLOWLY SLIDING DOWN YOUR SLIPPERY SLOPE?

For formerly traumatic dieters, their slippery slope's slow slide may be heralded by the almost imperceptibly gradual return of their hunger or cravings. If that happens to you, especially if you had managed to shut them down with your Reset and life thereafter, you may make the mistake of thinking that something inside you has changed. You may also be frustrated and terrified as a return to a life of lost dietary control raises the possibility that this time will be like every other time and that your weight's going to return. If you've had an easy time with hunger prevention and your cravings had diminished or disappeared only to return with a vengeance, the first thing to do is to check your food record to ensure that you're still practicing all of your cardinal hunger-prevention strategies.

More often than not, I'll see hunger and cravings return when one or more of those cardinal strategies slide; the most common cause of the slide is invariably the cessation of recording—which is almost always the first strategy to be let go. People may have been keeping records for months at a time, eating the same familiar meals and safe snacks, and have seen their weight consistently go down without any degree of suffering. In turn this leads a person to a sense of security, a sense that they've licked their problem, that they're cured. Their newly forged confidence then translates to their deciding that they're in control and consequently they no longer need to keep records.

For the first while after the cessation of recording they do just fine, but then slowly, sometimes over many months or even years, things start to change. The timing between meals and snacks becomes less uniform. Protein starts to disappear, first from the snacks and then often from breakfast. Breakfasts grow smaller. Snacks start to get skipped.

Really what's happening is that person is reverting back to their old habits, which while perhaps not conducive to successful weight management were and are extremely comfortable.

While there are certainly physiologic changes associated with weight loss that have an impact on things like metabolism, they generally don't suddenly heighten a person's appetite or generate cravings, especially not many months or years after a weight loss. If that's happening and you're not keeping a food record, resume immediately. If you're already keeping a food record, take a long look at it. Compare your recordings now with recordings you were making when things were easier. Has anything changed with your timing, your protein, or your minimums? If not, have you added or changed your exercise schedule? Have you changed jobs or are you working new shifts? Is there a new stress in your life? Are you sleeping well?

If after careful analysis you can't find any identifiable and correctable reason for the recurrence of your hunger or cravings, the next step would be to add some calories to your day. I usually encourage people to try to add them to their breakfasts and morning snacks. Start with an additional 100 calories a day and slowly add more if necessary.

YOU MUST BE THIS TALL TO EAT THIS MEAL

I remember when my wife and I were first married, she gained a small amount of weight. I wasn't involved in nutrition or weight management at the time, and I had only the most rudimentary understanding of things, but I figured that the crux of the matter was that my wife was matching my portions. She told me that she felt she deserved to eat as much as I did, and while I certainly didn't disagree (I've always known better than to ever do that), the simplest way to put it was that yes, she "deserved" to eat as much as me, but the amount of food I was eating supported *my* weight; if she ate the same amount as me, eventually perhaps she'd weigh the same, too—and I've got quite a few inches of height on her.

What I'm getting at, of course, is that the smaller you are, the tougher navigating our modern-day food environment will be. After all, there are no signs on a menu reading, *You must be this tall to order this meal.* Regardless of height, go out to eat and order the same item as your 6-foot-4 college football–playing son, and you'll both get served the same meal.

The only way to truly get a handle on your personal portion sizes is to have an idea of how many calories you ought to be aiming for per meal and snack, something you can easily calculate online at this book's website, TheDietFix.com. Once known, that will allow you to put portions into your own personal context.

READING IS MORE EFFECTIVE FOR WEIGHT LOSS THAN RUNNING

In an article published in the *Journal of Consumer Affairs*, Dr. Bidisha Mandal set out to determine the impact that food-label reading and exercise had on weight.[8]

She used data from the National Longitudinal Survey of Youth, which has followed 12,686 middle-aged men and women. Included in the survey were questions regarding the use of food labels, as well as questions regarding levels of physical fitness.

Dr. Mandal divided folks into those who read food labels always/often and folks who regularly participated in vigorous activity. She then further subdivided folks into those who were trying to lose weight, those who were trying to stay about the same weight, and those who weren't trying to do anything about their weight. Finally, she analyzed data from the 3,706 folks who between 2002 and 2006 consistently reported actively trying to manage their weight.

She then looked at four different subgroups:

1. Folks actively trying to manage their weight who neither read food labels nor participated in vigorous physical activity
2. Folks actively trying to manage their weight who read food labels and participated in vigorous physical activity
3. Folks actively trying to manage their weight who read food labels and did not participate in vigorous physical activity
4. Folks actively trying to manage their weight who did not read food labels but did participate in vigorous physical activity

Then using some fancy statistical analysis, she compared the impacts of label reading and vigorous exercise in various combinations on weight management. What she found was rather fascinating.

First, the expected: folks who were trying to manage their weight and read food labels and vigorously exercised were the folks who were the most successful.

Now the unexpected. Folks who were trying to manage their weight and who read food labels but didn't exercise were more successful than those who were trying to manage their weight who exercised but didn't read food labels.

Remember, your brain is more important than your brawn for weight management, and it's far easier to not eat calories than it is to burn them.

Knowledge is power.

Why Reading Food Labels Matters to Health

One of the largest drivers of diet-related chronic disease is misinformation, and the playing field we face as consumers in our supermarkets is anything but level, with food manufacturers enjoying a very unfair advantage.

With health claims, both overt and covert (implied), and governments that don't seem to care, consumers are left to fend for themselves in the face of the food industries' massive marketing machines. Let me give you an example: Chocolate Cheerios. The box tries to impress you with:

Whole Grain Guaranteed
Made with Real Cocoa
May Reduce Risk of Heart Disease

The website tries to bedazzle you with:

> *One delightful serving of Chocolate Cheerios® has 9 grams of sugar and*
> *is a heart-healthy choice for your whole family.*
> *Diets low in saturated fat and cholesterol may reduce the risk of heart*
> *disease.*

It sure seems incredibly healthy; it might even suggest to you that if you feed it to your family, they'll reduce their risk of heart disease. It's got to be a better choice for you and your children than the Froot Loops you grudgingly buy them, no?

No.

Let's compare the two. Spoon per spoon, yes, those "healthy" Chocolate Cheerios contain 20 percent less sugar and 2.5 percent fewer calories than Froot Loops, but they also contain 35 percent more sodium and 28 percent less fiber. So which do you choose?

If you're concerned about health, I recommend neither. But my guess is most consumers will automatically associate the Cheerios brand and the product packaging's claims as meaning the product's healthy and a slam-dunk better than Froot Loops. Except that they're not. Neither is a great choice. It's safest to never trust the fronts of packages, as the safest assumption is that if the packaging is trying to convince you that the contents are healthful, there's a better chance that they're not than that they are.

I'M HUNGRIER WHEN I . . .

Keeping a careful food record certainly allows you to identify patterns. Many women will notice that the week before their periods, they're hungrier. Shift workers will notice that different shifts have different impacts on their cravings and appetites. Hard-core fitness fanatics will find the type of exercise they do and its duration will affect both hunger and cravings.

Use your food records to look for these patterns and then to troubleshoot them.

For premenstrual hunger, up the calories during that week by 100 to 200, spread throughout the day and preferably in the mornings.

For shift work, there's likely to be some trial and error. Some shift workers struggle more the day after their shift change. Others struggle more the day of. Use your food record and keep track not only of what and when you're eating, but also the degree of your hunger and cravings, so that you can compare the patterns of easy, in-control days with those that are more challenging. Once you've identified the pattern, it'll be easier to attend to.

For fitness folks, while certainly you can work on fueling yourself properly for exercise, you may be well advised to also seek some advice from a dietitian with special interest in sports nutrition. The good news here is that the dietitian will have an easy time working with you as you'll bring to the table a detailed and carefully kept food diary.

FOOD ADDICTION: CHICKEN OR EGG?

Food addiction's a hot topic these days.

Proponents posit that food addiction is a real phenomenon that leads people almost irresistibly to eat. Opponents believe that it doesn't exist, and it's just a means by which people justify their difficulties with food. What if they're both right?

A recent study's got me thinking. Now, be forewarned, it's an animal study and therefore not necessarily transferable to human beings, but nonetheless . . .

The study looked at mini-pigs, in which brain activation of seven diet-induced obese mini-pigs was compared to brain activation of nine lean mini-pigs following an overnight fast.[9] The findings were striking. The obese mini-pigs had a great deal more activation of their brains' prefrontal cortices compared to the lean mini-pigs; the prefrontal cortex has been shown to be involved in addictive behavior in humans.

They also found decreased activation in the reward centers of the obese mini-pigs' brains. If in fact these results are applicable to humans, they suggest the possibility that so-called food addicts may be experiencing the phenomenon whereby food regularly consumed for its physiologic rewards (reducing stress, for instance) loses its ability to make them feel good over time. In turn, this might explain food addicts' requiring larger and more frequent quantities of indulgent foods to get their fix as well as why dietary restraint may be so difficult.

But here's the thing: the mini-pigs, with clearly different brain chemistries, didn't self-select for being obese; they were chosen by the researchers to be fed. At first they ate fairly normally, despite having ready access to food all day long (as opposed to their lean brethren). But over time, living in their all-you-can-eat buffet hutches, they started to eat more. By the end of the experiment, they weighed nearly double the weight of their peers. And by the end of the experiment, their brains had changed.

This may suggest that while food addiction indeed has neurophysiologic foundations, it's the chicken and not the egg. Meaning that these pigs weren't born addicted to food; they developed food addictions after living in what might be described as a toxic food environment.

That's exciting to me, in that if we can help people regain control over their food environments, if we can help people ease into more satiating patterns of eating, maybe we can rewire their brains, and in so doing, short-circuit these unnaturally derived neural pathways and responses.

And ultimately, I think we can. Why? Because I see it in my offices on a very regular basis. Though not every time, mind you—there are some folks who seem to truly struggle with these behaviors regardless of the tweaks we try. Which is why I think both proponents and opponents are right, that food addiction has a real physiological foundation, but that there is certainly a pattern of eating that may in some cases predispose people to heightened neurophysiological drives to eat.

Of course, when you think about it, none of this is particularly surprising. After all, couldn't the same thing be said about pretty much every addiction?

MOVE

Why exercise? As noted earlier, it's not because you're going to burn off your pounds; but at the same time, not exercising will decrease your likelihood of long-term weight management success. More important, though, not exercising will markedly impair your health, as without a doubt, exercise is the healthiest behavior you can possibly undertake. Its inclusion in your life will mitigate many of the theoretical risks your doctor may be ascribing solely to your weight. And if you don't overdo it, it can be a heck of a lot of fun.

ENCOURAGE YOURSELF TO EXERCISE

Let's face it, we all live pretty busy lives. Most people aren't going to rank exercise particularly highly if asked to rank the activities in their lives that they enjoy.

When it comes right down to it, people are consumers of time. If we're lucky, we might each find a few precious blocks of time a day when we're not working, tending to our families, eating, on the telephone, or sleeping. Those of us trying to include exercise in our lives somehow need to inspire ourselves to intentionally exercise during those few, fleeting free moments.

One way to encourage yourself to exercise more is to up the ante and make exercise more interesting by building in some rewards. Not food rewards, of course, but rewards that have value to you. Massages, books, time alone, spa visits, new clothing—whatever works for you. For rewards, first you'll need an exercise tracking system. It could be as simple as printing off a blank calendar and filling it with *X*'s on the days you exercise, or as complex as tracking your exercise on a website or smartphone app like Fitocracy (www.fitocracy.com). Feel free to visit my profile there at www.fitocracy.com/profile/yonifreedhoff. Regardless of your system, though, create a predetermined and quantifiable goal that once reached, earns you a reward. It's crucially important that you follow through with the actual reward rather than simply say you're going to; if you've mentally accepted that you probably won't end up treating yourself at the end of your hard work, you're going to be much less likely to do the work in the first place.

Remember, too, that the lengthy visit to the gym—the "pack your gear, get into the car, drive to the gym, hit the changing room, stand in line for equipment," and then do it all over again in reverse routine—just isn't going to happen most days for most people. To compensate for this, many people buy home gym equipment; they think that by having it at home, they'll be more likely to exercise. Yet what do most people do with those great intentions and new equipment? They banish them to their basements, out of sight, in a part of their homes that is often less than welcoming, and sometimes even beside the kitty litter atop a cold unfinished concrete floor.

If you want to actually use your home exercise equipment, one of the easiest ways to help yourself do so is to put it back into your line of sight. Seeing it may remind you first and foremost simply that it's *there*, and then also (potentially) of the money and good intentions that had you bringing it into your home. So if your home gym is hiding in the basement, consider relocating it to somewhere where you can see it, ideally somewhere you think it might be enjoyable to use, while staring out a window or at a television, whatever works. Alternatively, spruce up your basement gym area to make it more inviting.

If you choose to put it in front of a television, consider creating a rule that allows you to watch your favorite shows only while on the treadmill (never mind the speed, just get on it).

Bottom line: you should set out to create an environment that includes some measure of enjoyment in your exercise and an environment that increases rather than decreases the value of the time you spend doing it.

WHAT ABOUT BIGGEST LOSER–STYLE EXERCISE?

As far as rapid nonsurgical weight loss goes, there's probably no weight loss program more rapid than that of the television show *The Biggest Loser*, where it's not uncommon for contestants to lose upwards of 150 pounds at an average pace of nearly 10 pounds a week.

Is this a healthy way to lose? Should massive amounts of exercise be part of your strategy, even if just in the short run?

Don't do it. My admonition here isn't simply referring to the fact that the *Biggest Loser*–style approach is anything but realistic. After all, virtually no one in real life has the time to undertake the incredibly large amount of exercise, let alone experience the show's almost certainly severe degrees of stress, peer pressure, and dietary restriction, fostered by the team and the competitive nature of the show (in which the team who loses the least weight has a member voted off and the last man or woman standing wins $250,000). No, my worry has more to do with the impact of *Biggest Loser*–style weight loss on metabolism.

In an article published in the *Journal of Clinical Endocrinology and Metabolism,* Dr. Darcy Johannsen and colleagues studied the impact seven months of *Biggest Loser* weight loss had on the resting and total energy expenditures of 16 participants.[1] They used all the latest gadgets to do so, including indirect calorimetry and doubly labeled water. What happened? By Week 6, participants had lost 13 percent of their body weight and by Week 30, they'd lost an incredible 39 percent. More important, by Week 6 *Biggest Loser* participants' metabolisms had slowed by 244 calories per day more than would have been expected simply as a function of their weight loss, and by Week 30, by 504 calories more. What that means is losing weight *Biggest Loser*–style actually slows metabolisms down further than would be expected by losing in a less extreme fashion.

For the *Biggest Loser* participants, what this study suggests is that contestants on the show are burning almost a meal's worth of calories *less* per day than would be expected. Even more interestingly, the extra slowing found with *Biggest Loser* weight loss is absent with another category of rapid losers, bariatric surgical patients.[2] What this suggests is that there might be something uniquely risky to a person's metabolism to lose weight in true *Biggest Loser* style of intensive binge exercise coupled with dramatic dietary restriction. Slow and steady may indeed win this race.

The *Biggest Loser* study concludes:

> Unfortunately, fat free mass preservation did not prevent the slowing of metabolic rate during active weight loss, which may predispose to weight regain unless the participants maintain high levels of physical activity or significant caloric restriction.

Here's how I spell that out to the real world. While some contestants on *The Biggest Loser* will have new external motivators to maintain their extreme behaviors, such as new careers as spokespeople or fitness trainers, those who don't may be doomed by the show itself to regain their weight. The lifestyles promoted by the reality television show *The Biggest Loser* are only "realistic" to those whose livelihoods and/or fame depend on them.

Case in point? Take Erik Chopin. He was the winner of the third season of *The Biggest Loser*. He lost just over 200 pounds. A few years later he was on *Oprah* to talk about his massive regain. Think Erik dropped the ball? Not me. I think *The Biggest Loser* provided him with an unrealistic and potentially metabolically dangerous approach to weight management, and in the process, stacked his deck entirely against him—so much so that when chatting with Oprah about his regain, he recounted how just that morning he and his wife had hit the gym at 5:00 a.m., despite the fact that he reported that he doesn't particularly enjoy exercise.

Don't try to be a Loser. Don't expect a strategy that you don't enjoy to last. You need to find a lifestyle that you can honestly enjoy, and binge exercising likely isn't going to be a part of it. A small amount of daily exercise is going to have a much greater long-term impact than overdoing it for a few weeks or months—and then realizing you can't sustain it. Suffering from time to time, as you're about to read, might be all right, but regularly? It just won't last.

IS SUFFERING EVER A USEFUL STRATEGY?

Probably, but first a brief backstory to serve as an illustration.

When I turned 40, like many folks with momentous birthdays I decided to make some healthy living resolutions, and included among them was weight lifting. I'd been fair to middling at aerobic activities all my life, but had never really focused much on resistance training. The thing is, as far as health and aging goes, resistance training's probably king, and so . . .

For quite a while, it was a blast. Sure, there were days when I wasn't too keen, but once I saw the rapid progress that's often part and parcel of the early days with a new routine, it was easy to keep going. But there was this one Monday when I just didn't want to go. Of course, there had been days here and there when I hadn't fully felt like exercising, but that Monday was by far the worst. I was dreading exercising. I was tired, and the last thing I wanted to do was my weights. I procrastinated for nearly 10 minutes in my office and finally, grudgingly, headed to my gym.

The routine our fitness director, Kelly, had me on at the time was a pyramid. I had two groupings of five exercises, and I was supposed to run through each of the exercises three times in succession. By the end of the first set of the first two exercises in the very first grouping, I was already trying to rationalize either stopping altogether, or dropping it down to just two sets of each rather than three.

I didn't do that, however. I sucked it up and did it all.

And I'm not going to blow smoke and tell you I was so glad when I was done, that I felt great and alive, and so on. I actually felt pretty miserable.

The reason I pushed through wasn't that one day of exercise really matters in the grand scheme of things, but rather because I didn't have any good reason not to do it and I knew that if I gave myself permission for no particularly good reason to shirk my exercise, it'd be that much easier to give myself permission for no particularly good reason the next time.

Of course, sometimes there are great reasons not to follow through with various best intentions, plans, and resolutions. But when there's no good reason, and it's just you versus you, I recommend not giving yourself that proverbial inch.

But wait—haven't I been preaching this whole book that suffering is a terrible strategy?

Yes, but there's a difference. If every single time I headed to the gym I loathed it, that'd be a clear-cut sign that I'd better find myself another way to exercise. That'd be excessive, unsustainable suffering. On the other hand, if I generally enjoy it but here and there don't feel like doing it, that's a clear-cut sign that I'd better stay on top of myself, as follow-through and consistency are how habits are gained.

And it doesn't apply just to exercise; it applies to life in general. Our human nature can easily get the best of us, if we let it.

So whatever you're trying to accomplish, sometimes, for your greater good, it might be worth suffering through a rough day. Habits persist through thick and thin, but at their beginnings, sometimes you need to really muscle through the thins.

PLAN FOR INJURY

While it's paramount that you do your best to prevent an injury (not doing too much too soon, respecting your body and backing off when you hurt, ensuring your form is correct, etc.), and while I'm certainly not wishing one on you, chances are at some point one's going to happen. Given exercise's indirect benefits in cultivating healthy living behaviors as a whole, sometimes an injury is globally destructive. Take Brenda Mc-Inney, for example. Brenda's a blogging friend and she's also been extremely successful in her own healthy living journey. Since 2007 Brenda's lost 130 pounds following the guidance of Tosca Reno's Eating Clean diet. When I asked Brenda if she's had any setbacks over the past five years, she talked about her two injuries—one to her ankle and one to her back. Both times she gained 15 pounds before recognizing that her drop in exercise had led her to change and relax her eating strategies: "It was frustrating and I had to really focus on not going back to bad habits. I felt like I had taken a giant leap backwards."

Being injured might also heighten the role of food for comfort, so I encourage you to plan ahead. Here's what that planning might look like.

- Take stock of what food is in the house and make a shopping list to ensure that the best possible dietary options are on hand.
- Remember that food is at least 80 percent of the equation, so commit to even more careful record keeping.
- Do a back-of-the-envelope calculation of how many calories your exercise regime might have been burning. If you can get away with it, try to reduce dietary intake by that same amount but spread the reduction evenly across the entire day (but still make sure you're hitting your minimum meal and snack calorie requirements).
- Make an appointment to see a doctor or physiotherapist and formulate a treatment plan. Having a plan might serve as something of a surrogate—the pride you might take in actively pursuing your rehabilitation could serve as a substitute for the pride you felt exercising.
- If it's possible, use your injury as an opportunity to try something new. If suddenly you can't run, maybe you can try water aerobics or tai chi. If you've injured your upper body, maybe it's time to meet your local gym's Nautilus equipment. And if you can't think of an alternative, consider hooking up with a personal trainer to see if they might have some suggestions.

THINK

So much of healthy living and weight management is mental. The main reason is simply that change itself is difficult and consequently needs to be consciously and regularly fostered. Learning how to do so may require thinking about some things a little differently.

CHANGE YOUR INTERNAL SOUND TRACK

Internal sound tracks are our automatic thoughts that arise both unwittingly and unwillingly from the depths of our unconscious. In some senses they help to shape your identity and unfortunately, identities don't need to be positive in order to be internalized. We all have our own internal sound tracks and, more often than not, they're pretty darn negative.

Much of our automatic thoughts stem from our interpretations of those very same destructive questions we covered on Day 5 of your Reset. In a sense, they're those questions' automatic answers, and while asking different questions can certainly help to defuse a challenging situation, it may also be worth re-recording your automated answers.

The first step in recording a new and supportive sound track is actually taking the time to stop and listen to the one you've got. For at least a week, carry a small notepad, and every time you have a negative self-thought, pull out the notepad and write down the thought you had, the situation you were in, and, if you can untangle it, the question you asked yourself that led to your negative thought. This is actually more difficult than it sounds, as oftentimes the thoughts are brief and fleeting. When you do write it down, write only on the left half of each page, and be sure to include some of the background, too—what event led up to the thought, what were the resultant negative emotions?

Once you've collected what you feel are the bulk of your recurrent negative self-talking points, you'll need to carve out an hour or so to sit down and rewrite them. As this is an exercise in quiet introspection, it'd probably be best for you to be in a quiet environment—don't try to complete this part of the exercise while your world, children, and life are spinning around you. Instead, wait until you find a little bit of your own time, when and where you're not likely to be interrupted.

Your Current Sound Track	Your Desired Sound Track
I fail at everything I try to do.	*I did my best, and my best when I've missed a meal or a snack is different from my best when I haven't.*
[Following a moderate night binge episode, hated myself]	[Noticed on review of my day that I missed morning snack. Set up my cell phone with a special ringtone to remind me of my morning snack.]
I'm useless.	*If my lifestyle can't include occasional fast food or convenience, it won't be sustainable* or *While it's not somewhere I want to eat regularly, given I used to eat out every day the fact I still might here and there is so much better than before.*
[Following a trip to McDonald's, felt defeated]	[Used the experience to look up McDonald's nutritional information to determine my best options for the next time I find myself there.]
I really shouldn't eat this.	*Life includes chocolate—I just need to have the smallest amount that leaves me happily satisfied.*
[Contemplating chocolate, feeling anxious and scared]	[Can't forget to ask myself, *Is it worth it?* and *How much do I need to be satisfied?*]
I'm losing too slowly to ever succeed.	*Slow and sustainable is much smarter than fast and temporary* or *One pound a week over time will add up, and being in a hurry never worked before.*
[Following a half-pound loss over a week, feeling despair]	[Took a moment to remember all the times I've crashed my weight only to struggle and regain; remembered, too, that I need to like my life if I'm going to keep living this way, and while it may be slow, I don't feel like I'm dieting, but rather that it's a new lifestyle.]

When you're ready, your job is to fill in the right side of the page. Fill it in with the thoughts you feel you ought to automatically be hearing in place of your automated yet negative sound track, and be sure to include the facts that back up your desired assertions.

If you're having trouble with the rewriting, here's a trick. Pretend you're helping your best friend or closest relative with this exercise—he or she is reading you their negative automated thoughts and asking what you think they should be playing in their stead. The automatic thoughts we have for our loved ones are usually quite positive; pretending that you're working for those you cherish may help you with the frustratingly difficult exercise of learning to love, respect, and admire yourself.

Once you've come up with your preferred sound track, you might want to carry your list around, and when you notice you're lapsing into negative self-talk, pull it out and willfully play the sound track you've crafted. While it may feel artificial at first, the more frequently you consciously play your new records, the more likely your internal DJ will play them automatically.

DO YOU SUFFER FROM "GOOD LIFE SYNDROME"?

Here's another one you won't find in the medical textbooks, yet I see it all the time.

A patient comes to me wanting to lose weight. I go through a medical, diet, and lifestyle history and find out this person's eating out three or more times weekly, enjoys a glass of wine nightly with supper (and like me, they have large glasses and heavy hands), and vacations for four or more weeks of the year. They've got sincere desire to lose, yet no desire whatsoever to change their biggest-ticket weight loss items—eating out, drinking, and frequent travel.

It's tough to blame them, too. Oftentimes these folks are in their fifties, they've worked hard all of their lives, and they've finally carved themselves out enough time to enjoy some of the fruits of their labor.

They've got Good Life syndrome. They want to lose weight, but they're not willing to give up the lifestyle they've worked for so long to achieve. Of course, desire, willingness, and readiness for change are all very different things.

Does this sound like you? If you are struggling with Good Life syndrome, is there a way to live it at home? Where you spend your hard-earned dollars on the finest food money can buy, but foods that you and your loved ones could spend time thoughtfully transforming? You might join a local community shared agriculture (CSA) program that offers weekly baskets of heirloom organic vegetables. Perhaps you can explore your local butcher shops for free-range, grass-fed, antibiotic-free meats. There's a great saying to help inspire you to buy higher-quality ingredients: "Pay your grocer, not your doctor." In other words, live the good life, but live it healthfully.

HOW TO DEAL WITH A "FOOD COP"

Figuring out how to achieve your goals in the context of your life's various companions can sometimes be extremely tricky. What might sound easy or manageable on the page—like my telling you to eat more frequently, include more vegetables in your meal, take 15 minutes a few times a day to move your body—might get a lot harder when you take into account how the other people in your home and work environment might react.

Do you live with a "food cop"? Someone who's always watching what you eat and asking you questions like "Are you sure you should be eating that?" or "Why are you having that if you want to lose weight?"

While perhaps they're well intentioned—the only people on the planet who'd feel comfortable making those types of comments are our first-degree relatives (parents, siblings or spouses)—they're also the people most capable of pushing our buttons.

There may be a few rare individuals who respond well to having a food cop looking over their shoulder. But most people resent it, and given the source, may be inclined to oppositional defiance and think to themselves, *I'll show you how much of this I can eat!*

Sometimes it's even a food cop who's no longer living with you pushing your buttons. Oftentimes it's the memories of a childhood in which food was unfairly rationed or restricted that leads a person to struggle. Because after all, succeeding in limiting indulgences would in a sense be validating someone else's cruel words or behaviors.

Ultimately, the only question that I think a loved one should be asking of you if they know you're trying to make a lifestyle change, is, "Is there any way that I can help you, dear?," and they're allowed to ask that question once a week. Any more than that and they're likely to just be pushing your buttons—and have your buttons pushed enough and you may not want to succeed, as your success would in some way reward a behavior that you absolutely resent.

Please show this section to your food cop, as perhaps it will speak to them as well.

HOW TO DEAL WITH A "FOOD PUSHER"

Food pushers.

You know them; they're the folks who insist you take far more than you want. The folks who ladle out gigantic portions of everything, make a show of having everyone finish what's on their plate, and pressure you to take seconds of everything. Usually, they're not trying to sabotage your efforts, but it sure can feel that way if it's already a struggle to do the right thing.

But there are ways around this that don't involve embarrassing conversations, social faux pas, or uncomfortable situations. Here's my not-yet-patented three-step process.

Step 1: Blame your doctor (and here it's true if you think of me as an extension of your medical care) and tell your food pusher that your doctor is worried about your health, has given you very specific instructions for what you're allowed and not allowed, and has asked you explicitly to ensure that you always serve yourself.

Step 2: Take significantly less food than you actually want, especially the stuff you think you'll enjoy and want the most. (Yes, I realize this is going to upset your host, but read on!)

Step 3: When you've finished your purposely small portions, make a minor production with your host of how much you liked such and such and doctor be damned, would it be all right if you went back for seconds?

At the end of the meal? You're happy because you've controlled your portions, and your host is happy because their food was so good that you disobeyed your doctor's orders. Your host has also likely long since forgotten that you didn't take all that much to begin with.

Food pusher defused.

HOW TO DEAL WITH THE "YOU SHOULD STOP LOSING WEIGHT" SPEECH

In my practice, I'm fortunate to see a great many people lose a great deal of weight, and I've noticed two trends.

First, it's usually somewhere between a 15- and 20-pound weight loss that folks start noticing. But it's the second trend I want to talk about, the "you should stop losing weight" speech. If you lose enough weight, your friends, relatives, and/or coworkers will start telling you to stop.

In my experience the "you should stop losing weight" speech tends to start happening after a person has lost on the order of 15 to 20 percent of their original weight (for example, a 30- to 40-pound weight loss if your starting weight is 200 pounds). Whereby a friend, co-worker, or relative will tell you to stop. They'll do so despite the fact that you may still be healthfully losing weight, or still have weight-related impacts to your quality of life or health.

Sometimes they'll even come right out and say you don't look well.

I've got two theories about this. There's the less likely theory of jealousy, but honestly I don't believe that plays a big role for most folks. I think the more likely theory is that consciously or perhaps unconsciously, the evolutionarily ancient parts of our brains aren't comfortable with weight loss.

Many major and sometimes fatal illnesses have a wasting-away component to them, so I wonder if we as a species have it hardwired in us to recognize weight loss as a sign of illness. Many of us, too, have personally watched friends and relatives waste away; seeing a friend or a relative lose weight may trigger memories and emotions that are less than pleasant.

But as long as you are losing weight in a healthful, sustainable manner, and are seeing your doctor regularly to make sure that there is nothing wrong, you should keep doing what you're doing. Ultimately, you're going to have to ignore your in-your-face friends, but at least by reading this, you can start preparing for it and not be shocked or dismayed if and when it happens to you.

KEEP IT OFF

The most important thing to remember about maintenance: if you're doing things right, it'll be easier to keep it off than it was to lose it.

Ask anyone who has traumatically dieted and they're likely to tell you stories about all the diets they've done that "worked," yet all they've worked at was helping them lose the weight, not to keep it off.

Oddly, traumatic dieters may look back on extremely strict weight loss programs fondly. Programs that had no chance of long-term success, because they basically involved eating almost nothing and suffering through the hunger. Programs with 800 calories in all-liquid form. Programs that use things like vitamin or hCG injections as placebos to convince those desperate enough that there's some magic in them, that they'll help them lose, when really losing is just because that's what bodies readily do when they're given only 800 calories a day.

Every traumatic dieter knows that losing weight is easy; all you have to do is suffer. It's keeping the weight off that's difficult.

If you're Reset, weight maintenance should be easier than weight loss because if you're going about things properly, by the time you've finished losing the weight, you'll be fantastic at all of the behaviors you'll need to keep it off. Doing things properly means having been honest with yourself and living the healthiest life you can enjoy; eating the smallest number of calories you need to be happy; and exercising as much as you can enjoyably fit into your life. Sure, your losses will probably occur more slowly than with your more extreme efforts, but when you finish losing (and I define *finishing* as not losing any weight at all over a three-month stretch), all you'll have to do is keep on living the way you're living and the weight simply can't come back.

The only way to regain your weight is to lose your lifestyle. Think of weight as a chronic condition and your lifestyle as its treatment. As with any chronic condition, if you stop treatment, the condition comes back.

If you've been honest with yourself throughout this process, then the most difficult part would have been the first month. By the time you finish losing weight, keeping it off should take you minimal time and effort. Tracking calories should be nearly effortless. You'll have some system or shorthand to streamline record keeping, you'll know your foodscape's calories by heart, and you'll have a repertoire of meals and snacks that meet your caloric needs and goals. You'll have an enjoyable amount of exercise built in, and you won't have any forbidden foods or artificial caloric ceilings. You'll know how to indulge thoughtfully, and you won't get alarmed or beat yourself up if you happen to slip up from time to time.

LESSONS FROM THE NATIONAL WEIGHT CONTROL REGISTRY

As I know you know by now, the National Weight Control Registry has spent nearly two decades collecting data on individual weight loss masters, with the average registrant having lost 67 pounds and kept it off for five or more years.

While one thing's clear from the registry—there are many ways to lose weight—what's striking is how important just three commonalities are to keeping it off successfully. The good news is that your Reset has covered them all.

1. Caloric reduction: 98 percent of masters report modifying their diets in some way.
2. Exercise: 90 percent of masters do it, the vast majority by simply walking.
3. Breakfast: nearly 80 percent of masters have it.

It's important to note that the speed of loss varied dramatically among registrants, and certainly the registrants who came from my office's program didn't lose it in a hurry.

"CAN I EVER STOP KEEPING A FOOD DIARY?"

Maybe.

I say maybe because while some people are able to successfully abandon formal food diarizing, other equally successful people start down lifestyle relapse's slippery slope as soon as they stop recording.

If you'd like to try to stop, I suggest that you start weighing yourself daily. While you'll notice day-to-day fluctuations, what you're looking for is your baseline, because the scale also keeps track of calories. If you're eating more calories than you burn, then over time you'll gain weight; if you're eating less than you burn, over time you'll lose weight; and if you're eating as many as you're burning, you'll maintain your weight.

I encourage patients to weigh themselves daily if they'd prefer not to record, so long as their weights remain within three pounds from the weight they had when they put away their food record. If their weight does climb three pounds, that's their cue to pay more careful attention—still without recording—to their daily strategies. If weight climbs five pounds from their floor, I encourage pulling out the food record and reemploying all of the strategies that had been employed to get them there—food diarizing, weighing and measuring, the whole shebang—because if you don't nip your weight gain in the bud, it's liable to bloom. ⊚

To read more about some of the registrants and the specific struggles they've had to overcome, I recommend you read Anne Fletcher's *Thin for Life*, for which she interviewed a number of weight loss masters. The only caveat is that Anne's book was written during the height of the low-fat era of dieting and consequently there's an emphasis on low-fat eating as a strong determinant of success. Of course, as the years went by and low-carb diets became the rage, more and more registrants were enrolling in the registry after following a low-carb approach. As borne out by the medical literature, what matters isn't what approach you've adopted to cut your calories, just that you maintain that approach and, as a result, your weight for the rest of your life.

WEIGH

Scales. They're the bane of every dieter's existence, and as anyone who's struggled with traumatic dieting will tell you, bathroom scales are important enough to warrant their own chapter.

For traumatic dieters the scale can both give and take away; the traumatic dieter lives and dies by the scale. A day when it's down is a "good" day and happiness abounds. A day when it's up and suddenly the storm clouds circle.

SCALE ADDICTION

During weight loss efforts, traumatic dieters tend to weigh themselves many times per day. They start out weighing themselves stark naked before breakfast, and then again after workouts, before meals, and of course before bed.

I call this "scale addiction."

While scale addiction is certainly not a condition written about in medical textbooks, that doesn't make it any less prevalent or harmful. Scale addiction leads people to step on the scale multiple times a day, whereupon if the scale does not go down, or worse yet, goes up, mild to severe mental anguish ensues.

I've met many scale addicts.

They tell me that rationally, they understand that getting on the scale multiple times a day won't make any difference, that they know weight doesn't change that rapidly, but that they just can't help themselves.

Sometimes for those folks I recommend that they turn their scales over, take out the batteries, put tape over their solar strips, or better yet, move them to the trunks of their cars.

The thing is, scales can be truly frustrating devices because they don't simply measure caloric intake versus caloric expenditure. Scales also measure clothing, water retention, constipation, time of the month, and time of day differences.

Folks who weigh themselves frequently will know that weight fluctuates both day by day and within a day.

So for scale addicts out there, here are two things you need to know.

First, there are 3,500 calories in a pound. While bodies are not mathematical instruments whereby if you do or don't eat 3,500 calories, you'll see a pound change on the scale, bodies do obey the laws of thermodynamics. Weight is mass, and mass is energy. What does that mean? If you step on a scale on a Wednesday and it says you weigh three pounds more than you did on Tuesday, unless you consumed *at least* the caloric equivalent of 19 Big Macs more than you burned, the scale is weighing something other than your actual body weight.

Second, scales show the consequence and not the cause. What moves the number on the scale is not the act of standing on the scale, it's what you're doing and choosing to do and ingest during the times you're not standing on the scale. The scale will always tell you what you weigh, but it will never be able to tell you how you're doing. You need to determine how you're doing by evaluating what and how you're actually doing by asking yourself questions such as: *What have my dietary choices been like? How's my fitness? Am I being thoughtful? Am I organized and consistent?*

At the end of the day, it's your life that can change the scale, not the other way around.

My recommendations? During a weight loss effort, weigh yourself at most once a week, stark naked, before breakfast. Remember, too, if the weight surprises you, and if you're also keeping a food diary, you can double-check to see if the number makes sense. If you've gained a pound or two, but your diary says you're on track, the scale is probably weighing something that doesn't count. During a weight maintenance effort, weigh yourself daily and get to know your body's natural weight fluctuations. You might even want to track them for a little while on a spreadsheet, as many people, especially women with menstrual periods, have regular, recurrent fluctuations. More important, whether you're trying to maintain your weight or actively lose, use the scale to nip any weight regain in the bud by staying on top of it rather than letting it get out of hand—but be careful not to let yourself get seduced.

SCALE SEDUCTION

Scale seduction is often an insidious problem. You start your hard-core "diet" and begin to lose weight, and bolstered by the sweet somethings of losses the scale whispers in your ear, you slowly become more and more strict with your dietary and/or exercise regimes. Basically, watching those numbers go down seduces you into thinking you've found a long-term lifestyle, when in fact all you've really found is an increasingly strict diet.

Overly restrictive, undereating/overexercising diets, regardless of weight loss, are generally doomed to fail when you finally get sick of the restrictions you don't particularly enjoy. When does that happen? Usually, when the scale stops whispering sweet somethings.

Even when things are going great, don't fall into the trap of scale seduction. Remember, it isn't really about what you weigh; it's about what you're doing about what you weigh—a point even more important when applied to scale avoidance.

SCALE AVOIDANCE

"When I know I'm not doing well I can't even look at the scale, let alone weigh myself. When I walk into the bathroom I look anywhere but down."

Scale avoidance is exceedingly common in traumatic dieters because it tends to afflict people who believe weight management must involve strict control. Those folks often diet to the point of excluding food consumed for pleasure or comfort. And almost invariably, at some point they'll give up and indulge—often with binge-type consumption.

What happens next? Suddenly, the scale that they have been stepping on multiple times daily (due to their scale addiction) is no longer their friend. In fact, they want nothing to do with it. And what's led them to their newfound scale aversion? Usually, just a single indulgent episode, during which, mathematically, those same people probably didn't actually consume sufficient calories to truly cause their weights to climb. For instance, maybe they had a piece of chocolate cake at a party. Now, a piece of chocolate cake—even a rich, large, decadent, thick piece—probably doesn't even contain a quarter-pound of calories, yet it's often enough to trigger scale avoidance.

For some, scale avoidance lasts a day or two. For others it can be weeks and even months or years, and often scale avoidance goes hand in hand with giving up on many or all of their healthy living strategies, and in many cases regain of some, if not all or more, of their lost weight.

What a shame, right?

In fact, the scale isn't your friend *or* your enemy. The scale is just a tool that can provide you with another piece of information with which to help inform your decisions. So you should never, ever let the scale push you around. Remember, your life is dynamic and so, too, are your weight and your healthy living efforts. Sometimes life is worth more calories. Sometimes for good reasons, and sometimes not, but life and weight are certainly not going to be reflected in straight lines.

HOW TO USE THE SCALE TO YOUR ADVANTAGE

With all of these scale-related pitfalls, how do you use a scale in a way that avoids trauma and helps you in your weight loss efforts? It's not as straightforward as just standing on it.

First, if you're trying to lose weight, it's important to pause before you step onto the scale to ask yourself, *How do I think I'm doing?* After all, what does the scale know?

As mentioned, how you're doing depends on how you're living, and the scale frankly knows nothing about that. If you're happy with how you've been living and you feel that you're making the healthiest choices you can enjoy, even if the scale goes up, it shouldn't be allowed to take away your pride in your accomplishments.

So once you've decided how you're doing, go ahead and step onto the scale.

Before looking at the number, you've got to remember several things. First, scales measure a lot of extras: clothing (if you're wearing any), constipation (which can add up to two pounds), water retention (time of the month, salty meals, and sore muscles can each add up to a handful of pounds). Second, your scale doesn't know if you have had great reasons for consuming certain calories. Remember, celebratory and comfort foods are part of the human experience and are almost by definition indulgent.

Okay, so now you're looking at the number. If you're happy with it, step down and you're done.

If you're unhappy with it, there are only two questions you need to ask yourself:

1. *Am I doing something to address this frustrating number?*
2. *Is what I'm doing to address the number SMART?* (See discussion in Day 9.)

If the answers to those questions are "Yes," then there's nothing to worry about, even if the numbers are not doing what you want them to do today. Remember, the very act of a weight loss effort involves bringing the law of averages into play—meaning that some weeks you'll lose far more than you'd expect, and some weeks far less. At the end of the day, your key to success isn't a certain amount of loss per week; it's a consistent and sustainable lifestyle, one that reflects the best life that you can enjoy, and not the best you can tolerate. It's that attitude that you will get you to, and keep you at, your "best weight."

Returning to the second question you posed: *Is what I'm doing to address the number SMART?* Here it also needs to be sustainable. Again, this goes back to the idea of "best weight." If what you're doing to lose weight isn't sustainable, you're just wasting your time and you'd better figure out a different strategy of "doing"—or simply expect only temporary results.

The bottom line for scales: you may not love the number you see staring back at you—it may even be distressing to you—but if you're doing something about it, and you know what you're doing is sustainable, you're doing great.

WHAT ABOUT BODY FAT PERCENTAGE SCALES?

You've all seen them, and I'm sure many of you have them: the scales where you take your shoes off and magically the scale tells you your body fat percentage.

These scales work via bioimpedance analysis, which involves a small electrical current being passed through your body from foot to foot. The signal travels up through the various components of your body (fat, muscle, bone) and then back down again, and the time it takes is measured by the scale. Because the current passes more slowly through fat and bone than muscle, the built-in mathematical algorithms allow the scale to guesstimate the percentage of you that's fat.

Even a good body fat percentage scale will have an error range of at least 4 percentage points, and you can effect more error by varying your hydration level.

So why don't I like them? Wouldn't it be a good thing to know your body fat percentage?

What many folks don't know when buying a body fat percentage scale is that body fat percentages change often disappointingly slowly and frankly, aside from exercising and losing weight, there's really nothing extra for you to do to speed things up. There are no pills, potions, or exercises that will accelerate the loss of body fat any more than what your best efforts are already providing. Add in the wide range of error that these scales tend to have, and now you've got a tool in your bathroom with the potential of providing you with daily discouragement, utilizing a number about which you can't do anything specific to change. Not so smart.

SCALE HOLIDAYS

Sometimes I'll recommend that a person take a scale holiday. Traumatic dieters are often extremely attached to their scales emotionally and as a consequence the scale has the power to break them, even if they're doing great.

As noted before, sometimes you'll weigh more than how you're doing, and there are also times in life where weight probably ought not to be dropping (vacations, times of high stress, birthdays, etc.).

For folks who can't seem to break themselves from using their scales as the scales of judgment, I encourage them to take a four- to eight-week scale holiday. If you don't trust yourself to be able to resist the temptation to step on your scale during a scale holiday, I recommend that you grab it and put it in the trunk of your car. If you don't have a car, put it somewhere high enough so that in order to reach it, you'll need to pull out a stepladder.

A scale holiday by definition means that you don't weigh yourself even once during the specified time period. Instead, every time you have the urge to weigh yourself, take a moment and ask yourself, *How am I doing?* The answer shouldn't be based on whether you feel you've lost weight or if your clothing's looser. You should base your answer on whether you're adhering to your healthy living strategies.

One caveat, though: you shouldn't take a scale holiday unless you're keeping a careful food diary. In the absence of a food diary, the scale is the only thing that gives you any indication, over time, of whether you're eating more or less calories than you're burning.

IS IT A "PLATEAU" OR IS IT A "FLOOR"?

Does this sound familiar? You think you're doing everything right but the scale just isn't moving.

You've hit a "plateau."

Of course, physiologically, plateaus don't exist. If you eat fewer calories than you burn, you ought to be losing. If you're not, perhaps the scale is measuring constipation, water retention, or clothing. So if you're not losing, and it's not just a trick of the scale, either you're burning fewer calories than you think, eating more than you think, or some combination thereof.

There is, however, such a thing as a "floor."

As the body loses weight, it adapts and literally slows down your metabolism. Lose a great deal of weight, and despite it being entirely unfair, you're almost certain to be burning significantly fewer calories than when you started. Eventually, the calories your body is no longer burning due to these adaptations will equal the calories your new lifestyle no longer has you eating. At that point, you won't have hit a "plateau," you'll have reached your new equilibrium—your new floor.

If you've stopped losing weight, there are really only two questions you need to ask yourself:

1. *Could I happily eat any less?*
2. *Could I happily exercise any more?*

If the answer to both is "no," there's nothing left for you to do. If the answer is "yes," by all means tighten things up. Do remember, though, that if you can't happily eat any less and you can't happily exercise any more, then—guess what—you're probably not going to.

HEAL

Your health can affect your weight in numerous ways. Whether by means of medical conditions that make weight loss more challenging, or medications that lead to frank gains, it's important to explore some of the more common medical contributors to weight as well as if there's anything you can do to help reduce their contribution to your struggles.

SLEEP

Sleep's crucial to weight management. While you can certainly start your Reset even if you're not currently sleeping well, addressing your sleep issues may help you dramatically with your goals. Poor sleep will hamstring your energy, mood, and motivation, and from a weight perspective, will almost certainly add some pounds.

An unpublished study presented at the 2012 American Heart Association conference in San Diego detailed an experiment with 17 healthy young men and women. It was an 11-day study. For eight days the subjects were allowed their regular amounts of sleep, while for three days they were awakened 80 minutes earlier than their averages. The researchers tracked their caloric intake throughout, and the results were dramatic. On sleep-deprived days, study subjects consumed on average 549 more calories! That's a meal's worth! There are many theories about why this would be the case. One recent study demonstrated that the brain's reward center responded more dramatically to food when sleep deprived.[1]

Another found an association between sleep deprivation and increases in the hunger hormone ghrelin, with concomitant decreases in the fullness hormone leptin.[2] But regardless of the cause, the link between lack of sleep and increased weight is pretty much indisputable.

If you struggle with sleep, or if you simply never feel well rested, it may well be worth a chat with your physician about your options. Sometimes a person's sleep issues have to do with falling asleep, and here good sleep hygiene—literally how your room is set up, how you utilize your bed, and ensuring that you go to bed at the right time for you—can help a great deal (my favorite book on sleep hygiene is Peter Hauri and Shirley Linde's *No More Sleepless Nights*). Terminal insomnia, or difficulty staying asleep, often responds to medications, including a few that are nonaddictive and don't have the rebound effect of a bad night if you forget to take them. There are medications that can treat sleep interruptions such as having to get up to go to the bathroom, and others that may help quiet down the racing thoughts that prevent you from drifting back into slumber. And if your sleep issues relate to menopausal symptoms, there are also medications (including nonhormonal options) that can lend a hand.

Sometimes sleep can be impaired and you might not even know it. If you never feel well rested, even after what on the clock looked like a good night sleep, you might have a condition called "obstructive sleep apnea." Covered in greater detail later in this chapter, sleep apnea is a common and treatable problem that simple testing can uncover.

Don't overlook your sleep as playing a role in your efforts. Help yourself, or get some help, and get some better sleep!

FINDING ALTERNATIVES TO COMMON MEDICATIONS THAT CAN LEAD TO WEIGHT GAIN

First off, I should note that there's not always going to be an alternative medication. Sometimes the lesser evil is taking a medication that has no appropriate alternatives, even if it has the potential to cause some weight gain.

I cannot state this more clearly: if you're on any of the medications listed below, don't stop taking them, and don't use this section as a source of medical direction. There are risks to stopping some of these medications, and more important, there may be reasons that you're on them of which you're not necessarily aware. Sometimes drugs that can cause weight gain are in fact the very best and most appropriate choice. Instead, armed with the information you'll find here, make an appointment with your physician to discuss your care along with whether a weight-neutral alternative to common medications is appropriate for your particular case.

For ease, I've listed them according to the diseases they treat.

Diabetes

Any drug that increases insulin levels has the potential to cause weight gain.

Insulin

Individuals on insulin therapy are clearly taking a medication that increases insulin levels. Of all of the available insulin options (and there are many), the one that is least likely to cause weight gain is insulin detemir.

Sulfonylureas

This group includes glyburide, glipizide, gliclazide, glimepiride, tolbutamide, tolazamide, and chlorpropamide. These drugs help to control blood sugars by causing your body to produce more insulin. They're generally not recommended as a first-line single-drug therapy unless there are contraindications to the use of other medications. If you're on one of these drugs, it may be worth chatting with your physician to see if there are other options available to you.

It's important to note here that there's nothing wrong with the use of sulfonylureas, and often they are part of a multidrug regimen aimed at keeping the difficult-to-control diabetic away from the requirement of injectable insulin.

Meglitinides

These include repaglinide and nateglinide, and also enhance insulin secretion.

Dipeptidyl peptidase-4 Inhibitors

This group includes all of the drugs that end with "gliptin." They work by means of increasing the activity of incretins, which in turn serve to decrease the body's release of a hormone called glucagon and in so doing help to increase the body's release of insulin and increase the time food spends in the stomach. These drugs tend not to lead to sudden blood sugar lows. To date, these drugs have been shown to be relatively weight neutral.

Alternative Diabetes Drugs That Don't Increase Insulin Production

Biguanides

Here we're talking about metformin. It sensitizes your body to insulin, allowing you to secrete and use less of it. The advantages of using metformin aren't restricted just to its mechanism of action but also to the fact that taking it is associated with a small amount of weight loss and improvements in cholesterol, and it does not tend to put you at risk for the sudden lows that insulin-secreting drugs do.

Alpha-glucosidase Inhibitors

These include acarbose and miglitol, and aren't used all that frequently. They work by reducing the body's ability to absorb sugars by partially blocking an enzyme in the intestines. People don't usually love these medications, as they tend to lead to increased flatulence.

Thiazolidinediones

These include rosiglitazone and pioglitazone. While these drugs do in fact decrease insulin resistance, they are still associated with weight gain. Rosiglitazone was found recently to be associated with an increased risk of heart disease in some users, and its use is restricted in some countries, though it is still available in the United States. That risk was not found with pioglitazone.

Heart Disease, High Blood Pressure, and Angina

Beta-Blockers

Any of these blood pressure drugs ends in "lol." These are drugs that block the beta-adrenergic receptors to help control blood pressure. They can cause some fatigue and potentially lead to a significant amount of weight gain. One retrospective meta-analysis found that individuals placed on beta-blockers over time gained as much as 20 to 40 pounds.[3]

When I was in medical school, beta-blockers were a first-line option for treatment for all patients with high blood pressure, but since then that recommendation has changed. While still appropriate as a first-line treatment for some patients (usually people who have had heart attacks, have heart rhythm or rate control issues, or who are also migraine sufferers), if you're only on a beta-blocker solely for your blood pressure it's probably worth a discussion with your family physician about whether it would be appropriate for you to change over to a diuretic, an ACE inhibitor, or an angiotensin receptor blocker.

Calcium Channel Blockers

These include amlodipine, diltiazem, and verapamil. Often indicated for people with angina or rate control issues, calcium channel blockers are not likely to cause true weight gain but can cause fluid buildup in the legs. As a hiker, I can tell you, "a pound on the foot is like five on the back"; if you do have fluid buildup in your extremities, assuming there's no medical reason not to, it may be worth either a switch of medication, or if indicated, the addition of a water pill.

Mood Disturbances

Unfortunately, many of the medications used in helping manage mood disturbances can cause weight gain.

Antidepressants

It's the oldest generation of antidepressants that have the greatest impact upon weight. This would include the tricyclic antidepressants (TCAs) and the monoamine oxidase inhibitors (MAOIs). Common TCAs include amitriptyline, nortriptyline, imipramine, and clomipramine, while MAOIs are very seldom used anymore.

The next generation of antidepressants are the selective serotonin reuptake inhibitors (SSRIs) and the mixed serotonin-norepinephrine reuptake inhibitors. Anecdotally, many have the potential for weight gain.

In my clinical experience and in my discussions with other bariatric physicians, it would appear that those with the least impact on weight include citalopram, escitalopram, and sertraline. If you can trace back a significant weight gain with the initiation of a different SSRI than those listed previously, it may be worth discussing with your prescriber whether a swap is an option. Before you jump onto one of the three SSRIs I mentioned, however, you should know that another non-SSRI antidepressant, bupropion, is almost certainly weight neutral and may in fact help with weight loss. That said, bupropion would be contraindicated in people who have a history of seizures, liver disease, or anxiety states.

Newer antidepressants have also been shown to be associated with weight gain, with mirtazapine notably associated with dramatic gains.

Ultimately, the control of your mood disturbance is far more important than the potential weight gain associated with some of the drugs used for treatment.

Antipsychotics

This class of medication can lead to very dramatic weight gain. Common members of this class include olanzapine, risperidone, quetiapine, and haloperidol.

Two newer antipsychotics have been shown to have much lesser effects on weight, aripiprazole and ziprasidone.

Antipsychotics are appropriately prescribed as a treatment for psychosis and conditions such as schizophrenia, and certainly should never be stopped without first speaking to a physician.

Of late some physicians have been prescribing antipsychotics as a means of treating depression or even treating sleep disorders (see following). If your antipsychotic was started for one of these indications and you've gained weight, please make an appointment to discuss alternatives with your physician.

Mood Stabilizers

These drugs are often used in the management of bipolar depression. Lithium and valproic acid can both cause significant weight gain. Lamotrigine, on the other hand, does not.

Sleep Disorders

While most medications used in the management of sleep have no impact on weight, of late some physicians have begun prescribing antipsychotic medications to help with sleep. If you have been prescribed an antipsychotic as a sleeping aid, perhaps inquire about alternatives including the low dose use of the antidepressant trazodone.

You may also consider working on your sleep hygiene, as the routines associated with sleep and your bedroom can have a impact on both falling and staying asleep.

Autoimmune and Inflammatory Diseases

Often these conditions will require the use of steroids for treatment. While steroids can increase weight (and appetite), there are no weight-neutral alternatives. You should never stop steroids without consulting a physician because not only does their cessation risk the recurrence of the condition they're treating, but cessation carries with it risks of its own.

Cancer

Some chemotherapeutic regimens, notably those for breast cancer, can cause weight gain. I imagine that it goes without saying that the risk of slight weight gain is dramatically outweighed by the benefits of a remission of your cancer.

MEDICAL CONDITIONS THAT CAUSE WEIGHT GAIN DIRECTLY

There are many medical conditions that can have a negative impact on weight, and while a discussion of all of them is beyond the scope of this book, here are a few of the most common.

Obstructive Sleep Apnea

Sleep apnea is strongly associated with weight gain. It's also associated with an elevated risk of sudden death, daytime headaches, daytime sleepiness, high blood pressure, and leg swelling.

The treatment of sleep apnea is straightforward and does not involve medications. The most common treatment involves sleeping with a device called a CPAP or an APAP machine. By means of either continuous or variable pressure delivered through a soft, comfortable nasal or full face mask, these machines keep your airways open while you sleep, preventing dips in blood oxygen levels and eliminating the stress that sleep apnea puts on your body.

Another method of treatment, usually reserved for those who don't tolerate CPAP and those with only mild to moderate cases, involves the creation of a customized mouthpiece that serves to help keep the airways open.

Weight loss can treat and in many cases cure sleep apnea, but because the condition is also related to neck architecture, and not simply neck weight, weight loss does not always eliminate it.

While it may take a few weeks to get accustomed to sleeping with a CPAP or APAP machine, those few weeks are well worth it as treatment of sleep apnea not only has the potential of helping improve your weight, it's likely to restore your energy and decrease your risk of sudden death.

If you have ever been told that you stop breathing or gasp for air while sleeping, or that you snore loudly, or if you never feel well rested even after a lengthy night's sleep, I would encourage you to chat with your physician about being tested for sleep apnea.

Hypothyroidism

While there are many ways a person can develop hypothyroidism, the symptoms of the disease are the same:

- Fatigue and weakness
- Weight gain despite poor appetite
- Dry skin
- Intolerance of cold
- Hair loss (often including the outer third of the eyebrow)
- Initially heavy periods and later cessation of periods
- Constipation
- Difficulty concentrating and memory disturbance
- Impaired hearing

The likelihood of you having a thyroid condition significant enough to affect your weight in the absence of some or all of the other symptoms is quite low, and routinely having blood taken to check for your thyroid's status is not recommended.

Treatment is quite straightforward by means of thyroid hormone replacement, but generally weight loss does not reduce dose requirements.

Polycystic Ovarian Syndrome (PCOS)

PCOS is the most common female endocrine disorder and affects up to 10 percent of premenopausal women.

While it has yet to be determined whether obesity leads to PCOS or PCOS leads to obesity, weight and PCOS are linked, and the majority of women with PCOS have overweight or obesity.

The symptoms of PCOS include:

- Irregularly spaced, infrequent periods
- Infertility
- Male pattern hair growth and loss
- Acne

PCOS is also associated with an overproduction of insulin.

Treatment includes both weight loss and metformin. Both will help to reduce insulin production, and treatment often leads to a reduction in the symptoms of PCOS.

If you are a premenopausal woman with weight to lose who has irregularly spaced, infrequent periods, please speak to your doctor about the possibility of PCOS.

Menopause

If you've felt as if you've slowed down with menopause, you're probably right. Studies on menopause demonstrate that on average, women burn 200 fewer calories per day postmenopausally.[4] On an annualized basis, that may be as much as 20 pounds' worth. The other thing you might notice is that weight distribution changes; premenopausally if you gained weight it was distributed all over the body, but postmenopausally it tends to be right in that midsection.

What we don't yet know is whether menopause itself shuts down metabolism, or whether the symptoms of menopause shut it down. It's quite possible that sleep and mood disturbances combined with the stress of a major life change lead women to burn fewer calories. Consequently, I am rather aggressive in treating the menopausal symptoms of my patients in the hope that doing so will help decrease the impact menopause may have on their energy expenditures.

If you're struggling with menopausal sleep or mood disturbances, it may be worth a chat with your physician to explore your options. There are in fact medications aside from hormone replacement therapy (HRT) that can be used, and there are definitely also circumstances in which HRT's benefits outweigh its risks.

CAN HERBAL SUPPLEMENTS HELP?

There certainly are a great many products out there that suggest they're going to help you dramatically lose weight. If any of them were dramatically effective, your physician would be prescribing them and I certainly would not need to be writing this book. Worse than the overt fraud associated with many of these products is the fact that unbeknownst to those who are buying them, many are tainted with prescription weight loss medications that in turn carry with them risks.

Doctors don't look down their noses at natural products. The vast majority of the drugs being used today had some basis or are directly created from natural substances. Tamoxifen for breast cancer, for instance, is from the bark of the yew tree, exenatide for diabetes was derived from Gila monster saliva, while the common aspirin was originally extracted from weeping willows.

What doctors do look down their noses at is the sale of drugs—and anything you take to treat a medical condition is by definition a drug—that don't have behind them well-designed clinical trials that prove the drug is both safe and effective. Yes, it's possible that some of the products out there simply haven't been tested yet and may well be the holy grail of weight loss, but until they're tested and proven safe as well as effective, I'd caution against taking them.

The notion that everything natural is safe and good for us is a bizarre and flawed one. Tobacco is natural, so is arsenic, and certainly there are a great many mushrooms that grow in my yard that I wouldn't want to add to my salad. Before you take untested natural products, remember that they may have side effects, long-term consequences, or interactions with your other medications or medical conditions.

ARE THERE PRESCRIPTION WEIGHT LOSS MEDICATIONS?

The short answer is yes. The longer answer is that there currently aren't any magic bullets out there, and that even drugs with proven benefits in weight management won't do much in the absence of an organized plan to back them up.

It's also important to note that using, wanting, or needing a medication to help with weight management shouldn't be thought of as a personal failure. If you're doing everything in your power to realistically and enjoyably control your calories, and your weight is having a distinctly negative impact on your health or your quality of life, it may be worth considering a medication. Simply put, if the risk of your current weight is greater than the risk of taking weight loss medications, and you're currently living the healthiest life that you can enjoy, it's worth *considering* medications. Considering, of course, doesn't mean taking; it means learning enough about the risks and benefits of the medications to make an informed decision.

If you're interested in prescriptive weight loss medications, set up an appointment with your physician to discuss your options.

WHAT ABOUT WEIGHT LOSS SURGERY?

The most common misconception about surgery is that it's a cop-out, an easy way out for people who lack willpower.

That's not true.

If you have tried everything you could think of to lose weight, and for whatever reason—genetics, metabolism, psychology, learned behavior, coexisting medical problems, necessary medications—you couldn't lose, why wouldn't you consider a procedure that statistically is proven to prolong your life while significantly improving its quality, that cures many weight-related conditions? Of course, *consider* doesn't mean have the surgery, it just means consider, which means that you've done enough homework to make an informed decision. These days that homework will usually involve a great deal of web surfing. I think to truly be an informed decision, it also necessitates meeting and speaking with both bariatric surgeons and folks who've themselves had the surgery.

If after you've informed yourself you aren't interested, then definitely don't let anyone try to bully you into it. As a physician it's my business to do my best to ensure my patients are informed enough to make educated decisions, not to bully or push them into them.

In terms of when it's worth considering, again it's just about statistics. If the risk of the surgery is less than that of the weight, surgery's worth exploring. Currently, the most commonly accepted criteria for surgery are a body mass index greater than 40 or a body mass index greater than 35 with weight-related comorbidities like high blood pressure, sleep apnea, type 2 diabetes, or heart disease. Given the remarkable cure rates for type 2 diabetes associated with bariatric surgery, there's some push to lower the weight cutoff to a body mass index of 30 for type 2 diabetics.

There are different types of surgery, and they can be broadly broken down into restrictive surgeries and restrictive plus malabsorptive surgeries. The most commonly available options include:

Laparoscopic Gastric Banding

During this procedure, an adjustable silicone band is placed around the upper portion of the stomach, which effectively restricts intake by restricting the size of the stomach. The band can be tightened and loosened by means of either remote control telemetry, or a needle introduced into a port that's left just under the skin, to adjust the amount of saline solution in the band. This is a purely restrictive procedure.

A recent study was highly critical of gastric banding.[5] A group of 442 case-matched patients were followed for six postoperative years. Half received a gastric bypass (discussed below), and half, a gastric band. While early minor complications were higher in the gastric bypass group (triple the rate seen in banding), early major complications were similar. Aside from that, it's all bypass, with the bypassed patients enjoying quicker losses, larger maximal losses, and significantly better maintenance of losses.

How much better? After six years, for every failed gastric bypass, there were four failed lap bands (with failure determined by BMI greater than 35 or reversal of the procedure). For every long-term bypass complication, there were two lap band complications, and for every reoperation of a bypassed patient, there were two of lap banded ones.

Vertical Sleeve Gastrectomy

During this procedure, the greater curvature of the stomach is removed from the body, leaving an elongated, small stomach that preserves the pylorus, the lower valve of the stomach. This procedure is restrictive in that it reduces the size of the stomach. It also affects weight hormonally in that after surgery, the body produces less of the hunger hormone ghrelin. Compared with the other surgical procedures discussed in this book, long-term data are lacking, and while in the short term the procedure appears to be very successful, science has taught us not to assume anything. We need to wait awhile longer before we can confidently discuss long-term efficacy.

Roux-en-Y Gastric Bypass

Undoubtedly, this is the current gold standard of available bariatric surgeries. The procedure involves creating a very small pouch out of the upper portion of the stomach and then detaching the rest of the stomach, but not removing it from the body. The small stomach pouch is then reattached lower down along the small intestine, effectively bypassing a portion of the intestine. Because calories and nutrients are absorbed by the intestines, this bypass contributes to both weight loss and the risk of vitamin deficiencies, though the calorie malabsorption appears to be short-lived. Consequently, it necessitates lifelong vitamin supplementation and monitoring. The small pouch leads to dietary restriction, while the disconnect of the larger portion of the stomach leads to markedly decreased ghrelin production. Because the lower valve of the stomach is not part of the new dietary tract, a fair percentage of patients will develop a condition called dumping syndrome, in which the overly rapid transport of carbohydrates from the small pouch to the large intestine leads to osmotic fluid shifts into the intestines, causing them to stretch; this may result in cold sweats, stomach upset and pain, anxiety, and diarrhea.

Biliopancreatic Diversion with Duodenal Switch

Commonly referred to as a "DS," this procedure can be thought of as a more extreme gastric bypass, in that a great deal more of the intestines are bypassed. Another notable difference is that the stomach's pylorus is preserved. While this protects against dumping syndrome, the lengthy bypass leads to far more common and severe vitamin and protein deficiencies, necessitating more careful surveillance and vitamin supplementation. In Canada, this procedure is reserved for those in the most dire weight straits. The increased risks of the surgery and of long-term vitamin deficiency complications have convinced some Canadian health authorities that only those with body mass indices greater than 55 will see the risk of their weights outweighing the risks of this more involved surgery.

PARENT

You might not be alone in this journey, and with rapidly rising rates of childhood obesity and an environment that leads to weight gain as the default, learning how to extend your skills to your loved ones is crucial. It may even begin before they're born.

PREGNANT? YOU'RE NOT EXACTLY "EATING FOR TWO"

When I practiced more traditional family medicine and saw my pregnant patients, many rationalized rapid and extreme weight gains as a pregnancy rite of passage and not a worry because after all, they were "eating for two."

It's probably time to rethink those attitudes.

In 2010, a study was published in *The Lancet* that looked at a within-family comparison of pregnancy weight gain and baby birth weight.[1] The study was enormous in scope, capturing 513,501 women and their 1,164,750 children. The findings were pretty straightforward, too—babies of women who gained more than 50 pounds during their pregnancies were roughly 5¼ ounces heavier at birth than those of women who gained between 17 and 22 pounds. Moreover, compared to those gaining 17 to 22 pounds, the larger-gaining mothers were 1.7 times more likely to have a high-birth-weight baby, and those gaining more than 53 pounds were 2.3 times more likely to do so.

Doesn't sound like much, but there are some other things to keep in mind when considering the results.

Excessive pregnancy-related weight gain is a very real driver of sustained maternal obesity; that is, the women simply aren't able to lose all of their pregnancy-related gains (and often this occurs over multiple pregnancies). And bigger babies have been shown to be at greater risk of developing obesity as adults.

Why do bigger babies have a greater likelihood of turning out to be adults with obesity? The working theory in the paper is that the intrauterine environments of babies born to women with greater pregnancy weight gains are different, and that these differences have an impact on dietary behaviors over the child's lifetime—meaning that something happens in the womb that predisposes these children to greater weight-related struggles as adults. Of course, it's also possible that the dietary habits in homes of women who gain a dramatic amount of weight during pregnancy differ from those who don't, with those differences accounting for the impact on dietary behaviors over the child's lifetime. Either way one thing's for certain: pregnancy offers a wonderful opportunity to explore your diet and remember that the "two" you're eating for aren't exactly equal in size. Eating for 1.2 sounds about right.

HOW CAN I HELP MY CHILD WITH HIS OR HER WEIGHT?

I worry about treating children directly. I wonder how many traumatic dieters recall the first diet their parents put them on. Furthermore, I wonder what those first diets and pressures did to their self-esteem and their relationships with food and weight management.

With the possible exception of children who already have significant weight-related illnesses (type 2 diabetes, high blood pressure, fatty liver), I think children should be spared the pressure of trying to manage their weights. Instead I think the onus is on their parents to live the very lives they want their children to live. It's not the children who make the grocery store purchases, cook, pack lunches, decide on meals out, or act as role models for active lifestyles. It's you, their parents, and if you're worried about your child's lifestyle, first you probably ought to straighten up your own.

One way to teach children without putting the pressure of weight management on their too-young-to-process-it shoulders is to involve them in helping you with your struggles. But even then, I would discourage you from making it explicitly about your weight. Instead, explain to your kids that you've decided to put a stronger focus on your health. That you want to work on the foods you're eating and the activities you're enjoying to try to maximize your health, improve your quality of life, and lengthen your lifespan. Then ask your kids for help.

While older kids may see right through this plan (though that shouldn't stop you from trying it out on them), younger kids will be absolutely thrilled to be involved, and in so doing you can help teach them about healthy living and eating without making it about *them*.

Some things you might do with your children?

- Spend an afternoon at a bookstore perusing different healthy cookbooks and choose a few that have recipes the kids themselves seem interested in.
- Make one night a week a family cooking night where either as a group, or one-on-one, you spend time with the kids cooking a healthful recipe. While you're cooking, you can discuss what it is about the recipe that you like, in terms of both preparation and health, and in so doing, give your children the incredible gift of being able to fend for themselves in a kitchen.
- When going through recipes, explain to your kids what you're looking for in a healthier recipe. Then talk about how to identify some options that fit the bill.
- Ask your children to help you find and try out some healthful snacks—ones with not too much in the way of calories and that also include protein. Once you've found some that you and your children like, ask them to help you to keep track of whether you've had your snacks between meals. Doing this will teach them the importance of between-meal snacks when it comes to sustaining daily energy levels and in preventing hunger.
- Consider hiring your kids as your own personal trainers—literally. Not only will they be thrilled to boss you around a gym; they'll be

there, too, and you can easily and nonoppressively create a "you only get paid if you do it, too" rule. If you don't want to go the money route, or if your kids are young enough to still enjoy spending time with you, just ask them to head out with you on walks, runs, cross-country ski trails, and the like.

- Sign yourself and your kids up for some local road races. They're great fun, and having something to train for will likely inspire both you and your children to pay more attention to food and fitness without weight being the focus.

Of course, if your child truly is suffering with weight, either directly as a consequence of a weight-related medical condition or indirectly as a consequence of something else, don't enroll them in any formal weight management plan or program before checking it out yourself first *without them*. You need to evaluate it from their eyes and from a nontraumatic dieting perspective to see if it's a safe place for them to turn to for help.

ARE YOU SETTING YOUR KIDS UP FOR A LIFETIME OF DIETARY STRUGGLES?

Are you catering to a picky eater at home? Do you make multiple short-order dinners? Do you cook the same bland kid foods over and over again? I feel your pain. We've got three little girls, and I know how frustrating it can be when kids turn up their noses at healthy meals. I also know about the anxiety felt when kids seemingly aren't eating anything. I've spent a fair bit of time reading the medical literature on healthy eating and I've learned from it that if there's a food they reject, the best way for us to get them to eat it is to try, try, try, try, try (and add a whole pile more tries) again.

Our home's rule is simple. You have to eat one bite of anything that's put on your plate. If you don't like it after a bite, you don't need to have more, and there are always a few different choices per meal (but second meals aren't prepared to replace wholly rejected first ones). My oldest probably took 30 runs at green leafy salads until she started eating them without pause. My middle kid, 30 runs at sweet potatoes. And the baby? So far she still eats pretty much anything.

Apparently, kids' palates are rather plastic, and just as I tell my girls, if you try a food enough times, eventually your tongue will learn to like it. Well, one day I got to thinking. I wondered if my palate's got any plasticity left? Can adults retrain their tongues to like new foods? To test it, I chose coffee.

Once upon a time, I had been a classic Canadian double-double drinker. What that means is that in my coffees I would have two creams and two sugars. By med school I'd swapped cream out for whole milk but had stuck with the sugar. Opening up my current practice I swapped down to skim milk and Splenda, but I never could go straight black. I tried here and there, but I found black coffee to be more than repulsive. I found it bitter, angry, and at clear odds with my tongue. Given that I drink coffee daily, usually two cups, I figured that I should use hideously black coffee to test whether I could retrain my taste buds.

July 29, 2011, was the day I started the experiment. I suffered through two vile black coffees daily for a few weeks. Then, somehow, they went from being absolutely vile to just being bad. A week later, and suddenly they were tolerable. And as I sit and type now, I'm enjoying my black coffee greatly.

Sixty cups of coffee was what it took to retrain my palate. In sips I estimate that represents 1,800 "trys."

So where am I going with all of this?

If our children grow up in homes where their palates are trained to enjoy highly processed, highly salted, nutritionally bereft boxed foods, take-out meals, and restaurants, what chance do you think they'll have at retraining their palates as adults to enjoy more healthful fare?

Wouldn't it be easier to train your kids' palates right from the get-go, setting them up for lifelong dietary success with constant and regular introductions of healthy foods, rather than take the processed and restaurant way out and set them up for a potentially lifelong dietary struggle?

I sure think so.

ARE YOU FEEDING YOUR CHILDREN PROPERLY?

Here I'm not talking about nutrition; I'm talking about how you actually feed them. What are your practices surrounding food? Do you have regular mealtimes? Do you use coercion to try to inspire vegetable consumption? Do you reward with treats?

Parental feeding practices have been the subject of a great deal of research, and in November 2011, the *American Journal of Clinical Nutrition* published a handy summary of it all.[2]

Here are the study's top 10 take-home messages:

1. Pressuring kids to eat fruits and vegetables and markedly limiting their access to sweets and fatty snacks, along with using food as a reward, are all strongly linked with out-of-control children's eating patterns.
2. The more inconsistent parents are with eating schedules or with serving healthy versus unhealthy foods, the worse it makes the first issue listed.
3. Having at least one parent at the family meal means children eat more fruits and vegetables, and are less likely to skip breakfast.
4. Adopting a knee-jerk pattern of dietary restriction with an overweight child may drive that child to be more, not less, likely to overeat.
5. The availability and exposure to foods at home most certainly affects children's long-term food selections and preferences.
6. The earlier and more broadly a child is exposed to different foods, the healthier that child's eventual adult diet.
7. The more fruits and vegetables you have available at home, the more fruits and vegetables your kids will eat.
8. The more fruit juice and breakfast bars you have at home, the less actual fruits and vegetables your kids will eat.
9. The more often meals are eaten in front of the television, the less often the family sits down to eat together, and/or the more food is used as a reward, the more your kids will drink sugar-sweetened beverages.

And number 10? I'll quote directly from the paper, as it pretty much sums up everything else up: *"Children like what they know and eat what they like."*

So to make sure your children know what healthy eating is, here are some straightforward prescriptions for healthy home eating:

- Encourage a wide and varied healthy diet, introducing new foods frequently and early.
- Don't pressure your children to eat (one-bite rules are fine) or withhold dessert unless they eat their veggies.
- Don't serve dessert every night.
- Don't reward them with food.
- Disband the "clean your plate" club.
- Keep plenty of fruits and vegetables handy, accessible, visible, washed, and ready, and actually smile at your kids when you or they eat them.
- Sit at the table and eat with your kids.
- Don't skip meals.
- Dramatically minimize restaurant and take-out meals.
- Ensure that as many meals as possible a week involve the transformation of raw ingredients (not mixing boxes).
- Involve your kids in cooking.

Or put even more simply: live the life you want your children to live.

AT LEAST ONE NIGHT A WEEK, SKIP AFTER-SCHOOL ACTIVITIES AND COOK

There's no debate, exercise is the single most important modifiable determinant of health. The even better news is that there's really no need for skill—plain old walking works great. Of course, that doesn't stop any of us parents from schlepping our kids here there and everywhere for exercise "lessons"—soccer, hockey, skating, dance—the list, and the time involved, can sometimes feel endless.

But with all of those after-school sports, is something else suffering? It sure looks that way, with one recent study revealing that kids who played more after-school sports were also consuming more sugar-sweetened beverages and fast food than their less-involved friends.[3] That same study also determined that after-school sports did not demonstrate any benefit in preventing childhood obesity.

What might be lost with all of these after-school skill-building activities? The likelihood of parents teaching their children the single most health-conferring skill imaginable: the skill involved in transforming raw ingredients into food. The skill of cooking.

Cooking is quickly becoming a lost art.

With the incredibly fast pace of our lives and the world these days, it's no wonder cooking's falling by the wayside. Between chauffeuring kids to their various after-school activities and the electronic tethers we all now wear, time has become more pressured than ever. And of course restaurants of all sorts are everywhere to fill the void.

But resistance isn't futile.

Resolve to ensure you teach your children how to cook—and if you yourself don't know how, this is your opportunity to ask them to help you to learn.

Find a simple and easy-to-follow cookbook that also includes nutritional information, then formally protect and conscript one night a week as a family cooking night. Each week, a different family member takes a turn picking, prepping, and cooking a recipe. Ensure that you schedule a time to shop for the recipe's ingredients before the day of, and perhaps even prep the ingredients together the night before cooking so that putting things together the next day is a quick snap. (Of course, parents can and should help—this isn't about division of labor; this is about sharing and learning the love and joy of cooking.) Then eat it together at the dinner table.

Your kid missing one extra after-school activity or not playing soccer particularly well isn't likely to have any negative long-term impact on their health. But their leaving your home not knowing how to cook will, as not only will it lead them into the processed food world's nutritionally terrifying embrace, it might lead them to lead their future families into it as well.

WHAT ABOUT SCREEN TIME?

There's no doubt whatsoever: screen time is associated with increased risk of obesity. What's fascinating, though, is that the risk isn't inactivity causing kids to burn fewer calories—it's that screen time leads kids to eat more of them.

Looking at television viewing, researchers in Greece found that while the kids who watched the most television were the heaviest, that relationship persisted even after they controlled for physical activity levels.[4] In the end, the researchers concluded that the kids who watched the most television were eating the most calories.

How or why does screen time lead to more calorie consumption? We don't know. Perhaps it's the fact that television commercials regularly show images of highly palatable food, and studies on seeing images of highly palatable food suggest that when we do see them, we eat more. Or perhaps it's something else entirely, as might be suggested by a very cool small study out of Denmark and Canada.[5]

Researchers took 22 healthy, normal-weight male teens and put them in two separate experimental settings. In the first, they played a seated hour of video games and then ate lunch. In the second they simply sat for an hour before eating. In each setting, the teens were allowed to eat as much lunch as they wanted.

When they played the video games, they burned more calories than they did just sitting (about 20 calories more), but on average they also ate 80 more calories at lunch. The kids denied feeling any hungrier, and they didn't compensate for the increase in lunch calories by eating fewer calories later in the day.

So why does video game playing cause increased calorie consumption? Who knows? The researchers in this study speculated that perhaps it either interferes with the body's ability to feel full post play or affects the players' brains' reward systems in some strange way, priming them to eat more.

Whatever the cause of the increased intake, it's another blow to the generally accepted notion that screen time causes weight gain because it keeps kids from being active. That's not to say that decreasing your children's screen time won't help with their health or weight, just that it's more likely to help by decreasing the calories they consume than by increasing the calories they burn.

You might also want to rethink your family's source of television signal. A recent study published in the Journal *Pediatrics*[6] revealed that while hours watching television were associated with increased weight in children, the association was significant only when the children reported "paying primary attention" to the programming. While researchers aren't entirely sure why attentiveness affected weight, one of the theories they put forward was that attentive television watching had child viewers seeing and internalizing more in the way of food commercials. If this were true, an easy workaround would be to consider a switch to a streaming media service such as Netflix. Not only will that cut out the commercials, but it'll also cut down on costs, as Netflix is far and away cheaper than even the most basic cable packages.

Based on this research, my advice to parents is straightforward. Rather than set up a lot of rules on amounts of screen time, set up three simple rules around food and screen time:

1. Kids should be allowed only healthful snacks while playing video games, surfing the net, or watching television. Generally, that means fresh fruit and vegetables—definitely no sugared beverages and no juice.
2. Create a system whereby meals don't immediately follow screen time. Perhaps set up a system whereby chores occur specifically in the 30 minutes before dinner.
3. Cut your cable and switch to a commercial-free streaming service like Netflix.

DOES EXER-GAMING COUNT AS EXERCISE?

The short answer is no.

Studies on exer-gaming's ability to burn calories have been underwhelming to say the least. Some studies have demonstrated that the actual calories burned during exer-games are negligible,[7] that it would take 60 hours of play to burn a single pound worth of calories.[8] Others have revealed that though utilized when first purchased, exer-game systems tend to collect dust over time.[9]

It's too bad, too—those games are an awful lot of fun. They're just not exercise.

Epilogue

Maryanne's traumatic dieting had her believing that she was too weak-willed to enjoy the foods that she found most comforting and rewarding. Consequently, she believed that for her, life couldn't include chocolate, among other foods. Slowly, Maryanne learned to trust herself, and while she never did feel comfortable enough to have boxes of chocolate sitting in her cupboard, she regularly visits her local corner store, which happens to sell a wide variety of 100-calorie chocolate bars. She'll even get full-sized bars from time to time. Most important, she no longer lets chocolate make her feel guilty.

Corrine and her husband had a few frank discussions and slowly he let go of trying to control her eating. At first, even though she knew he was trying, his every glance during mealtimes caused her blood to boil. But slowly, she learned not to care. Corrine worked through Thomas Cash's *The Body Image Workbook*. When she decided to take a weekend dance class and her husband didn't join her, she signed up with her best friend. Corrine's now a size 12, a proud, happy, and healthy size 12. She and her husband are in counseling, and while she hopes they'll work things out, she's ready for whatever her future has in store for her.

Eunice took quite a while before she was finally able to let go of her decades of traumatic dieting. She joined and left my office's program seven times before finally admitting to me that when she left the office, she'd always go right back to her mental games around perfectionism, would weigh herself six times a day, and would deny herself any food that she didn't feel fit in a diet. Letting go of all of that, she actually started to lose. At the age of 66, with two arthritic knees, and being only five feet tall, her loss sure hasn't been in a hurry. Here's hoping she sticks with it and doesn't let her traumatic dieting demons get the best of her.

Julie took her improved mood onto the dating circuit and near the beginning of her weight loss journey met a man who didn't care one bit about her weight. She admits that finding someone who loved her at her higher weight in a sense reduced her desire for weight loss and that perhaps that's why she's going out to eat a bit more frequently than her weight would like. But then she laughs and says that she's going out to eat the smallest number of times that she needs to enjoy her life.

George struggled with losing weight. One day he came to me and told me that he was embarrassed to have to do so, but he wanted to talk about bariatric surgery. I reassured him that there was nothing to be embarrassed about and that his job was to do his best. If his best still left him with diabetes and an impaired quality of life consequent to his weight, then that surgery was a real option. Currently, George is on the waiting list for a gastric bypass.

Steven has yet to come back to my office. Maybe one day he'll be ready for slow and sustainable, or perhaps he's conquered his weight on his own. Here's hoping he's happy and healthy.

Karen eventually got pregnant without the help of the fertility doctor. She never did lose the full 100 pounds she was told she needed to lose, but far more important, she learned how to use food to keep herself in control of her eating urges, and in so doing, stopped her psychologically devastating binge eating.

Weight loss is a personal journey. There's so much more to it than simply eating less and exercising more. While you're going to have a great many ups and downs in life, and however you decide to lose or maintain your weight, here are the 10 things I don't want you ever to forget:

1. If you can't happily eat any less, you're not going to eat any less.
2. If you can't happily exercise any more, you're not going to exercise more.
3. If you don't like the life you're living, you're not going to keep living that way.
4. If you accept your personal best at everything else in life, you probably should for your weight, too.
5. If you can't use food both for comfort and celebration, then you're on a diet that you're ultimately going to quit.
6. Simply tolerating your life isn't good enough.
7. There are some things in your life affecting your weight that you're not going to be able to change.
8. Your best weight is whatever weight you reach when you're living the healthiest life you actually enjoy.
9. The more weight you'd like to permanently lose, the more of your life you'll need to permanently change.
10. Reality isn't reality television, and it most certainly does include chocolate.

There's absolutely no doubt in my mind that you *can* transform your life and that this time *will* truly be different. This time you're going to do *your* best, not the best there is, and *your* best changes day by day, hour by hour, and minute by minute, and not only includes but embraces imperfection. It's this recognition—that your best is dynamic—that will help you to get back on the horse when you inevitably get thrown off. And it's this recognition that will afford you the ability to not just live your life, but to love it. You're here on this planet once and you owe it to yourself to ensure that you like your life while you're here. Improving your health may require changes, and while there's not yet a way for you to get a new deck, stacking the one you've got doesn't need to be a misery. Yes, there'll be effort required, but if there's regular suffering, you're doing something wrong. You're aiming for the healthiest life that you can enjoy, not the healthiest life that you can tolerate. Given that the crux of all of this is truly and honestly liking your life, there's no reason whatsoever for even one moment to think this can't be done. You *can* do this, and without suffering, there's truly nothing stopping you.

NOTES

Preface

1. Canadian Obesity Network, *Obesity Status Report,* Leger Marketing, February 22, 2011, p. 22.
2. Vetter MI. What do resident physicians know about nutrition? An evaluation of attitudes, self-perceived proficiency and knowledge. *Journal of the American College of Nutrition.* 2008:**27(2)**:287–298.
3. Kruger J et al. Dietary and physical activity behaviors among adults successful at weight loss maintenance. *International Journal of Behavioral Nutrition and Physical Activity.* 2007:**3**:17.

Dieting's Seven Deadly Sins

1. Pelchat ML. Images of desire: food-craving activation during fMRI. *Neuroimage.* 2004:**23(4)**:1486–1493.
2. Baumeister RF et al. Ego depletion: is the active self a limited resource? *Journal of Personality and Social Psychology.* 1998:**7405**:1252–1265.
3. Shiv B, Fedorikhin A. Heart and mind in conflict: the interplay of affect and cognition in consumer decision making. *Journal of Consumer Research.* 1999:**26(3)**:278–292.
4. Westerterp KR, Speakman JR. Physical activity energy expenditure has not declined since the 1980s and matches energy expenditures of wild mammals. *International Journal of Obesity.* 2008:**32**:1256–1263.
5. Luke A, Dugas L, Ebersole K, Durazo-Arvizu RA et al. Energy expenditure does not predict weight change in either Nigerian or African American women. *American Journal of Clinical Nutrition.* 2009:**89(1)**:169–176.
6. Pontzer H, Raichlen D, Wood B, Mabulla A et al. Hunter-gather energetics and human obesity. *PLoS One.* 2012:**7(7)**:e40503.

Dieting's Seven Deadly Traumas

1. Foster G et al. What is a reasonable weight loss? Patients' expectations and evaluations of obesity treatment outcomes. *Journal of Consulting and Clinical Psychology.* 1997:**65(1)**:79–85.
2. Yanovski SZ. Binge eating disorder: current knowledge and future directions. *Obesity Research.* 2003:**1**:306–318.

Post-Traumatic Dieting Disorder

1. Domoff SE et al. The effects of reality television on weight bias: an examination of *The Biggest Loser. Obesity.* 2012:**20(5)**:993–998.

The Mythology of Modern-Day Dieting

1. Flicker L, McCaul K, Hankey G, Jamrozik K, Brown W, Byles J, Almeida O. Body mass index and survival in men and women aged 70 to 75. *Journal of the American Geriatrics Society.* 2010:**58(2)**:234–241.
2. Kuk JL, Arden CI, Church TS, Sharma AM, Padwal R, Sui X, Blair S. Edmonton Obesity Staging System: association with weight history and mortality risk. *Applied Physiology, Nutrition, and Metabolism.* 2011:**36**:570–576.
3. Rampersaud E et al. Physical activity and the association of common FTO gene variants with body mass index and obesity. *Archives of Internal Medicine.* 2008:**168(16)**:1791–1797.
4. McTiernan A et al. Exercise effect on weight and body fat in men and women. *Obesity.* 2007:**15**:1496–1512.
5. Polivy J. Psychological consequences of food restriction. *Journal of the American Dietetic Association.* 1996:**96(6)**:589–592.
6. Pittler M, Ernst E. Dietary supplements for body-weight reduction: a systematic review. *American Journal of Clinical Nutrition.* 2004:**79(4)**:529–536.
7. Harp J. Obesity in the National Football League. *Journal of the American Medical Association.* 2005:**293(9)**:1061–1062.

Day 1: Gear Up!

1. Hooper L, Summerbell CD, Thompson R, et al. Reduced or modified dietary fat for preventing cardiovascular disease. *Cochrane Database of Systematic Reviews.* 2011:**7**:CD002137.
2. Willett WC, Skerret PJ. *Eat Drink and Be Healthy.* New York: Free Press: 2005.

Day 2: Diarize!

1. Hollis JF et al. Weight loss during the intensive intervention phase of the weight-loss maintenance trial. *American Journal of Preventative Medicine.* 2008:**35(2)**:118–126.
2. Lally P et al. How are habits formed: modelling habit formation in the real world. *European Journal of Social Psychology.* 2010:**40(6)**:998–1009.
3. Champagne CM, Bray GA, Kurtz AA, Monteiro JB, Tucker E, Volaufova J, Delany JP. Energy intake and energy expenditure: a controlled study comparing dietitians and non-dietitians. *Journal of the American Dietetic Association.* 2002:**102(10)**:1428–1432 PMID: 12396160.

Day 3: Banish Hunger!

1. Wyatt HR, Phelan S, Wing RR, Hill JO. Lessons from patients who have successfully maintained weight loss. *Obesity Management.* 2005:**1**:56–61.

Day 6: Exercise!

1. Jakicic JM et al. Effect of exercise on 24-month weight loss maintenance in overweight women. *Archives of Internal Medicine.* 2008:**168(14)**:1550–1559.
2. Jakicic JM et al. Prescribing exercise in multiple short bouts versus one long continuous bout: effects on adherence, cardiorespiratory fitness, and weight loss in overweight women. *International Journal of Obesity and Related Metabolic Disorders.* 1995:**19(12)**:893–901.

Day 8: Eat Out!

1. Mayer J et al. Accuracy of stated energy content of restaurant foods. *Journal of the American Medical Association.* 2011:**306(3)**:287–293.

Reset Any Diet

1. Groves B. William Banting, father of the low-carbohydrate diet. Weston Price Foundation. Available at: www.westonaprice.org/know-your-fats/william-banting-father-of-the-low-carbohydrate-diet. Accessed March 30, 2012.

2. Banting W. *Letter on Corpulence Addressed to the Public.* 4th ed. London: Harrison, 1869.

3. Mente A et al. A systemic review of the evidence supporting a causal link between dietary factors and coronary heart disease. *Archives of Internal Medicine.* 2009:**169**(7):659–669. Siri-Tarino PW et al. Meta-analysis of prospective cohort studies evaluating the association of saturated fat with cardiovascular disease. *American Journal of Clinical Nutrition.* 2010:**91**(3):535–546. Hooper L et al. Reduced or modified dietary fat for preventing cardiovascular disease. *Cochrane Database of Systematic Reviews.* 2011:7:CD002137.

4. Weigle DS et al. A high protein diet induces sustained reductions in appetite, ad libitum caloric intake, and body weight despite compensatory changes in diurnal plasma leptin and ghrelin concentrations. *American Journal of Clinical Nutrition.* 2005:**81**(1):41–48.

5. Low-carb bubble about to burst? CNN Money. Available at: http://money.cnn.com/2004/03/19/news/companies/lowcarb_overkill/index.htm. Accessed March 30, 2012.

Eat

1. Barr S, Wright J. Postprandial energy expenditure in whole-food and processed-food meals: implications for daily energy expenditure. *Food and Nutrition Research.* 2010:**53**. DOI: 10.3402/fnr.v54i0.5144.

2. Magnuson BA et al. Aspartame: a safety evaluation based on current use levels, regulations, and toxicological and epidemiological studies. *Critical Reviews Toxicology.* 2007:**37**(8):629–727.

3. European Commission Health and Consumer Protection Directorate-General, Scientific Committee on Food. Opinion of the Scientific Committee on Food: update on the safety of aspartame. SCF/CS/ADD/EDUL/222. Final. 2002. Available at: http://ec.europa.eu/food/fs/se/sef/out155_en.pdf. Accessed March 30, 2012.

4. Gardener H, Rundek T, Markert M, Wright C, Elkind M, Sacco R. Diet soft drink consumption is associated with an increased risk of vascular events in the Northern Manhattan Study. *Journal of General Internal Medicine.* 2012. DOI: 10.1007/s11606-011-1968-2.

5. Phelan S, Lang W, Jordan D, Wing R. Use of artificial sweeteners and fat-modified foods in weight loss maintainers and always-normal weight individuals. *International Journal of Obesity.* 2009. DOI: 10.1038/ijo.2009.147.

6. Blackburn GL et al. The effect of aspartame as part of a multidisciplinary weight-control program on short-term and long-term control of body weight. *American Journal of Clinical Nutrition.* 1997:**65**(2):409–418.

7. Spill M, Birch L, Roe L, Rolls B. Hiding vegetables to reduce energy density: an effective strategy to increase children's vegetable intake and reduce energy intake. *American Journal of Clinical Nutrition.* 2011. DOI:10.3945/ajcn.111.015206.

8. Mandal B. Use of food labels as a weight loss behavior. *Journal of Consumer Affairs.* 2010:**44(3)**:516–527.

9. Val-Laillet D, Layec S, Guérin S, Meurice P, Malbert CH. Changes in brain activity after a diet-induced obesity. *Obesity.* 2011:**19(4)**:749–756. PMID: 21212769.

Move

1. Johannsen DL, Knuth ND, Huizenga R, Rood JC, Ravussin L, Hall KD. Metabolic slowing with massive weight loss despite preservation of fat-free mass. *Journal of Clinical Endocrinology and Metabolism.* 2012. DOI: 10.1210/jc.2012-1444.

2. Das SK, Roberts SB, McCrory MA, Hsu LK, Shikora SA, Kehayias JJ, Dallal GE, Saltzman E. Long-term changes in energy expenditure and body composition after massive weight loss induced by gastric bypass surgery. *American Journal of Clinical Nutrition.* 2003:**78(1)**:22–30. PMID: 12816767.

Heal

1. St-Onge MP et al. Sleep restriction leads to increased activation of brain regions sensitive to food stimuli. *American Journal of Clinical Nutrition.* 2012:**95(4)**:818–824.

2. Taheri S et al. Short sleep duration is associated with reduced leptin, elevated ghrelin, and increased body mass index. *PLoS Medicine.* 2004:**1(3)**:e62.

3. Lee P. Metabolic sequelae of β-blocker therapy: weighing in on the obesity epidemic? *International Journal of Obesity.* 2011:**35(11)**:395–403.

4. Lovejoy JC et al. Increased visceral fat and decreased energy expenditure during the menopause transition. *International Journal of Obesity.* 2008:**32(6)**:949–958.

5. Romy S., Donadini A, Giusti V, Suter M. Roux-en-Y gastric bypass vs gastric banding for morbid obesity: a case-matched study of 442 patients. *Archives of Surgery.* 2012. DOI: 10.1001/archsurg.2011.1708.

Parent

1. Ludwig DS, Currie J. The association between pregnancy weight gain and birthweight: a within-family comparison. *Lancet.* 2010:**376(9745)**:984–990. DOI: 10.1016/S0140-6736(10)60751-9.

2. Scaglioni S et al. Determinants of children's eating behavior. *American Journal of Clinical Nutrition.* 2011:**94(6)**:2006S–2011S.

3. Nelson TF, Stovitz SD, Thomas M, LaVoi NM, Bauer KW, Neumark-Sztainer D. Do youth sports prevent pediatric obesity? A systematic review and commentary. *Current Sports Medicine Reports*. 2011:**10(6)**:360–70. PMID: 22071397.

4. Manios Y, Kourlaba G, Kondaki K, Grammatikaki E, Anastasiadou A, Roma-Giannikou E. Obesity and television watching in preschoolers in Greece: The GENESIS Study. *Obesity*. 2009:**17(11)**:2047–2053. DOI: 10.1038/oby.2009.50.

5. Chaput JP et al. Video game playing increases food intake in adolescents: a randomized crossover study. *American Journal of Clinical Nutrition*. 2011:**93(6)**:1196–1203.

6. David S. Bickham, Emily A. Blood, Courtney E. Walls, Lydia A. Shrier, and Michael Rich, Characteristics of Screen Media Use Associated With Higher BMI in Young Adolescents, *Pediatrics* 2013; **131:5** 935–941; published ahead of print April 8, 2013, doi:10.1542/peds.2012–1197.

7. White K et al. Energy expended by boys playing active video games. *Journal of Science and Medicine in Sport*. 2011:**14(2)**:130–134.

8. Graves L et al. Comparison of energy expenditure in adolescents when playing new generation and sedentary computer games: cross sectional study. *British Medical Journal*. 2007:**335**:1282.

9. Owens SG et al. Changes in physical activity and fitness after 3 months of home Wii-Fit use. *Journal of Strength and Conditioning Research*. 2011:**25(11)**:3191–3197.

Recipes

I can't say that I subscribe to any particular dietary modality. I'm an equal opportunity eater. The recipes that follow are truly the recipes from my home kitchen. Tested, tweaked, tuned, and written up here by my wonderful wife, they won't suit everyone, but they may be a starting point for folks who are embarking on new experiences in cooking. I'm also not suggesting that these are the world's healthiest recipes—just that my family likes them and that my wife graciously agreed to write them for the world to see.

Some of these recipes contain artificial sweeteners—as mentioned earlier in the book, I'm not worried about their consumption, but if they worry you, feel free to substitute the sweetener of your choice in its equivalent amount (though this might affect cooking and consequently you might need to tweak the recipe some). Many folks who are reticent to use artificial zero-calorie sugar substitutes are comfortable using stevia, a plant-based zero-calorie sweetener that's available in any health food store. You'll also notice some recipes that call for whey isolate protein powder. We'll often use flavored powders. I don't feel strongly about one sort of protein powder being better than others—though there are certainly some people who do. Last, we also use those low-fat options whose tastes we don't mind. No worries if you want to use full-fat versions; just recalculate the calories.

Calorie and protein calculations were done using *Mastercook 9.0*'s database and our home's stock ingredients. While our numbers can guide you, to be accurate it'd be best for you to recalculate (for example, a slice of our bread may differ in calories from a slice of yours).

Between the breakfast and lunch/dinner recipes, there are snack suggestions that may fall just shy of this book's protein recommendations. In that case, you may need to either slightly increase the portions or combine snacks together. I'll often have them alongside some nuts or cheese.

BREAKFASTS

Yoni's "Be Prepared to Share" Smoothie

Yoni has been having this smoothie for breakfast at least five mornings a week for the past eight years. It's called "Be Prepared to Share" as it's a rare morning when one of our three daughters doesn't nab some from him. If you don't have Swiss chard, feel free to substitute spinach or kale, and if you're looking for an alternative to frozen berries, frozen mango works well.

Servings: 1 | Time to Table: 2 minutes | Can be made the night before, then reblended quickly out of the refrigerator

½ cup pasteurized egg whites
½ cup skim milk
½ cup fruit-flavored low-fat Greek-style yogurt
1 extra-large banana

¼ cup old-fashioned rolled oats
1 cup frozen berries
3 large leaves Swiss chard, with stems

Combine everything in the blender and blend!

Per serving: 476 calories, 35.7g protein

If the calories are too high for you, omitting the oats will bring them down to 381 and the protein to 32.2g.

Baked Apple Cinnamon Oatmeal Crisp for the Oatmeal-Fatigued

Servings: 6 | Time to Table: 40 minutes | Freezable

Canola oil cooking spray

2 cups old-fashioned rolled oats

¼ cup loosely packed brown sugar

2 teaspoons ground cinnamon

1 pinch salt

1 teaspoon baking powder

6 tablespoons whey isolate protein powder (often a level scoop, but double-check your brand; I use a vanilla ice cream–flavored one)

1 large or extra-large egg, or ¼ cup pasteurized egg whites

1½ cups skim milk

⅓ cup unsweetened applesauce (about the size of a single-serve portion)

1½ tablespoons unsalted butter, melted

1 teaspoon vanilla extract (optional)*

2 medium apples, peeled, cored, and chopped (I like Empire, but Spartan, McIntosh, or Granny Smith do well, too)

Preheat the oven to 400°F and spray a 2-quart oblong ovenproof glass baking pan with cooking spray.

In a large bowl, combine the oats, brown sugar, cinnamon, salt, baking powder, and protein powder.

In a separate bowl, combine the egg, milk, applesauce, butter, and vanilla. Add to the dry mixture and mix well.

Combine the apples with the wet mixture.

Pour into the baking pan and bake for 25 minutes or until set. Remove from the oven, let cool slightly, and cut into 6 servings.

Per serving: 287 calories, 15g protein

*If using vanilla-flavored protein powder, I leave out the vanilla extract.

Quick and Hearty High-Protein and Flax Oatmeal

Servings: 1 | Time to Table: 5 minutes | Freezable in muffin tins

⅓ cup old-fashioned rolled oats

2 tablespoons whey isolate protein
   powder (I use the vanilla flavor)

1 tablespoon ground flax seeds

⅔ cup skim milk, plus more if
   needed

1 tablespoon unsweetened
   applesauce

½ teaspoon ground cinnamon

1 teaspoon brown sugar

Combine the oats, protein powder, ground flax, and skim milk in a microwave-safe bowl. Stir and place in the microwave oven on high power for 3 to 4 minutes, stirring every minute, until cooked.

Remove from the microwave and stir in the applesauce, cinnamon, brown sugar, and protein powder. Add more milk as needed.

Per serving: 306 calories, 21g protein

High-Protein Whole Wheat Berry and Buttermilk Pancakes
(aka Homemade Toaster Pancakes)

The best part about these pancakes is that if you make extra, you can freeze them. Then when you're in a rush, throw them in your toaster and away you go. You can use strawberries, mixed frozen berries, or baked apple slices in place of the blueberries.

Servings: 4 (3 pancakes each) | Time to Table: 20 minutes | Freezable

1 cup buttermilk (shake well
   before measuring)

1 cup light sour cream

1 large egg

2 teaspoons vanilla extract

¼ cup vanilla-flavored protein
   powder

1 cup whole grain whole wheat
   flour

2 tablespoons sugar

1 teaspoon baking powder

1 teaspoon baking soda

¼ teaspoon salt

1 cup blueberries

1 teaspoon unsalted butter

Syrup, for serving

Combine the buttermilk, sour cream, egg, and vanilla in a small bowl and mix well. Sift the protein powder, flour, sugar, baking powder, baking soda, and salt together into a large bowl. Fold the wet ingredients into the dry, doing your best not to overmix (it should be a bit lumpy). Fold the blueberries into the batter.

Heat up a large pan over medium heat and grease it with the butter. Place approximately ⅓ cup batter per pancake in the pan, leaving 2 inches between each pancake. Cook until bubbles start to form on top, then flip. Cook for another minute or two. When both sides are golden brown, remove from the pan. Add maple syrup at 55 calories per tablespoon or a light syrup for about half that (27 calories per tablespoon). Keep in mind that there is already a bit of sugar in the recipe, so these pancakes really don't need much syrup at all.

Per 3-pancake serving: 300 calories, 15g protein (not including syrup)

Homemade Egg-and-Cheese on an English Muffin

A slice of tomato and some pepper often show up in mine.

Servings: 1 | Time to Table: 5 minutes

1 whole grain whole wheat English
muffin

1 ounce part-skim or light
mozzarella cheese, thinly sliced
1 large egg

Cut the English muffin in half and top with the cheese. Toast in the toaster oven. Cook the egg in a nonstick pan, flipping once after 1 minute. Place the cooked egg in between the two halves of the English muffin and enjoy!

Per serving: 336 calories, 24g protein

Anyone Can Cook Two-Egg Cheese Omelet with Tomato, Onion, and Mushroom

Feel free to omit or exchange any of the listed veggies, or add to them. And don't be scared of greens—chopped cooked spinach or Swiss chard makes a nice addition to any omelet!

Servings: 1 | Time to Table: 10 minutes

2 large eggs

2 tablespoons skim milk

Freshly ground black pepper

Canola oil cooking spray

2 teaspoons chopped onion or shallot

1 medium white mushroom, chopped

2 or 3 cherry tomatoes, chopped

1 ounce low-fat cheddar cheese, thinly sliced

1 slice whole grain whole wheat bread, toasted

Beat the eggs in a bowl with the skim milk. Add black pepper to taste.

Spray a small pan with cooking spray. Add the onions and mushroom and cook until tender, about 1 minute.

Add the cooked vegetables and tomatoes to the egg mixture. Pour everything back into the pan and return the pan to the heat.

When the eggs look solid around the edges, add the cheese to one half of the omelet. When the cheese is mostly melted, fold one half of the omelet over the other half. Remove from the pan and enjoy with the slice of toast!

Per serving (including toast): 297 calories, 24g protein

No Excuses Two Eggs, Any Style, with Whole Wheat Toast

Why does it need to be complicated? Make sure you calculate any additional calories if using any spreads on the toast. If you're looking for a substitute for the toast, try a sliced avocado with a touch of salt, pepper, and a drizzle of high-quality olive oil and fresh lemon juice.

Servings: 1 | Time to Table: 5 minutes

2 large eggs
Salt and freshly ground pepper,
   optional

Smoked paprika, optional
2 slices whole grain whole wheat
   bread, toasted

Cook the eggs in any style you like (scrambled, over easy, sunny-side up, poached, hard- or soft-boiled, etc.). Season with a bit of salt and pepper to taste, or with smoked paprika if you're so inclined. Enjoy with the whole grain whole wheat toast.

Per serving: 296 calories, 18g protein (not including any spreads)

Stupidly Easy Homemade Whole Wheat Crêpes

These crêpes can be used to make Apple Cheddar Crêpes (recipe follows), yogurt berry crêpes (add plain fat-free Greek-style yogurt and berries to the middle of the finished crêpes), peanut butter banana crêpes (spread peanut butter and sliced bananas down the middle of the finished crêpe), or cheese blintzes (see page 282). Crêpe batter can also be frozen in individual portions for use at a later date.

Servings: 7 (1 crêpe each) | Time to Table: 20 minutes | Freezable (batter)

1 large egg
1 teaspoon vanilla extract
1 teaspoon canola oil
1 teaspoon baking powder
¾ cup whole grain whole wheat
   flour

1 cup skim milk, plus more if
   needed (batter thickens while
   sitting)
Canola oil cooking spray

In a medium bowl, beat the egg with the vanilla, canola oil, and baking powder. Let stand for 1 minute and then remix. Beat in the flour and milk. Mix well, removing as many lumps as possible.

Let the batter sit for 5 minutes to remove air bubbles. (You may need to add a small amount of milk to the batter, a tablespoon at a time, if it appears too thick or is not spreading well when poured into pan.)

Heat a medium nonstick frying pan over medium heat and spray it lightly with cooking spray. When the pan is hot, ladle in approximately 3 tablespoons of batter, tilting the pan to evenly coat the bottom.

When the edges begin to curl off the pan, use your fingers to pull the crêpe up from the pan and flip it over. Cook for another 30 to 40 seconds on the other side before removing the crêpe. Repeat until all the batter is used up, making 7 crêpes.

Per plain crêpe: 77 calories, 4g protein

Amazing Apple Cheddar Crêpes

Servings: 4 | Time to Table: 10 minutes

1 recipe Stupidly Easy Homemade Whole Wheat Crêpes (page 280)
1 large apple (I like Granny Smith or Empire, but feel free to use your favorite)
1 teaspoon ground cinnamon
5¼ ounces low-fat cheddar cheese
Canola oil cooking spray
7 teaspoons maple syrup

Prepare the crêpe batter.

While the batter is sitting, core, peel, and thinly slice the apple. Place in a microwaveable bowl and sprinkle with the cinnamon. Microwave on high power for 1 to 3 minutes, until soft, stopping once to stir.

While the apple is cooking, cut the cheddar cheese into thin slices.

Heat a medium nonstick frying pan over medium heat and spray it lightly with cooking spray. When the pan is hot, ladle in approximately 3 tablespoons of batter, tilting the pan to evenly coat the bottom.

When the edges begin to curl off the pan, use your fingers to pull the crêpe up from the pan and flip it over. Add ¼ of the cheese, placing it down the middle of the crêpe in a single row, then place ¼ of the apple slices on top of the cheese. When the cheese begins to melt, fold one side of the crêpe into the middle, then fold in the other side of the crêpe over the top of the first folded side.

Remove from the pan and top with 1 teaspoon maple syrup. Enjoy!

Per 2-crêpe serving: 288 calories, 18g protein (including syrup)

Holy Moly Cheese Blintzes

If you're uncomfortable with the Splenda and low-sugar jam, feel free to use stevia or sugar, but of course that will change the calories.

Servings: 3 to 4 | Time to Table: 30 minutes

Canola oil cooking spray

1 pound low-fat, low-sodium, pressed (dry) cottage cheese

2 large eggs

3 tablespoons Splenda

1½ teaspoons fresh lemon juice

1 teaspoon vanilla extract

2 tablespoons skim milk

1 recipe Stupidly Easy Homemade Whole Wheat Crêpes (page 280), cooked

Low-sugar jam, for serving

Low-fat sour cream, for serving

Prepare the crêpe batter. Preheat the oven to 375°F and spray a large ovenproof glass baking pan with cooking spray.

Combine the cottage cheese, eggs, Splenda, lemon juice, vanilla extract, and milk in a food processor and blend until smooth.

Place ⅓ cup (85g) of the cottage cheese mixture in the center of each crêpe. Fold one side of the crêpe into the middle, then fold in the other side of the crêpe over the top of the first folded side. Place the blintzes side by side in the baking pan and bake for 20 minutes. Serve topped with low-sugar jam and low-fat sour cream.

Per 2-blintz serving: 344 calories, 39.2g protein (not including toppings)

SNACKS

Soy Pumpkin Muffins

I use silicone mini muffin pans for these. To freeze, place the muffins in a heavy-duty resealable plastic bag. Then pop one into the microwave for a few seconds to thaw and reheat.

Servings: 28 (1 mini muffin each) | Time to Table: 30 minutes (plus cool down) | Freezable

3 cups soy flour	½ teaspoon ground ginger
2 cups Splenda	4 large eggs
2 teaspoon baking soda	⅔ cup water (or more if batter is
¼ teaspoon salt	too thick)
1 teaspoon ground nutmeg	½ cup canola oil
2 teaspoons ground cinnamon	½ cup unsweetened applesauce
½ teaspoon ground cloves	2 cups canned unsweetened
½ teaspoon ground allspice	pumpkin puree

Preheat the oven to 350°F.

With a fork, stir together the flour, Splenda, baking soda, salt, nutmeg, cinnamon, cloves, allspice, and ginger in a bowl. In another bowl, combine the eggs, water, canola oil, applesauce, and pumpkin puree.

Fold the wet ingredients into the dry, doing your best not to overmix (it should be a bit lumpy). Divide the batter equally in muffin pans, 3 tablespoons for each muffin. Bake for 20 minutes or until a toothpick inserted in the center of a muffin comes out clean. Let cool for a few minutes in the pan, then pop out and store in a tightly closed container.

Per muffin: 93 calories, 7g protein

"Creamy" Lemon-Cranberry Soy Muffins

I use silicone mini muffin pans for these. To freeze, place the muffins in a heavy-duty resealable plastic bag. Then pop one into the microwave for a few seconds to thaw and reheat.

Servings: 18 (1 muffin each) | Time to Table: 40 | Freezable

Canola oil cooking spray

2 cups soy flour

1 tablespoon baking powder

¼ teaspoon salt

Grated zest and juice of 1 lemon

½ cup Splenda

¼ cup sugar

1 cup skim milk

1 large egg

1 cup unsweetened applesauce

2 teaspoons canola oil

⅓ cup water, plus more if needed

1 cup fresh or frozen cranberries,
    cut into halves

Preheat the oven to 400°F and spray a silicone mini muffin pan with cooking spray.

In a large bowl, mix the flour, baking powder, and ¼ teaspoon salt together with a fork. In a separate bowl, combine the lemon zest, Splenda, and sugar. Add to the flour mixture.

In a small bowl, combine the lemon juice and milk. Let sit for a few minutes (it will look curdled, but that's okay). With the fork, stir in the egg, applesauce, canola oil, and water.

Make a well in the dry ingredients and pour in the wet ingredients. Stir with the fork until evenly moistened, then fold in the cranberries. If batter is too thick, add small amounts of water until it reaches the consistency of brownie batter.

Divide the batter evenly in the muffin pans, 3 tablespoons per muffin. Bake for 30 minutes or until a toothpick inserted in the center of a muffin comes out ever so slightly moist and the tops are slightly browned. Let cool for a few minutes in the pan, then pop out and store in a tightly closed container.

Per muffin: 79 calories, 7g protein

Aviva Heller–Style High-Protein
Banana Oatmeal Chocolate Chip Muffins

As a grade school boy, Yoni had a best friend whose mother used to make oatmeal chocolate chip muffins that to this day Yoni still speaks highly of. While these aren't her exact recipe, they were made in her and her muffins' very fond memory. I use regular or mini silicone muffin pans for these. To freeze, place the muffins in a heavy-duty resealable plastic bag. Then pop one into the microwave for a few seconds to thaw and reheat.

Servings: 8 regular to 16 mini (1 muffin each) | Time to Table: 35 minutes | Freezable

Canola oil cooking spray

3 large ripe bananas

¼ cup Splenda

2 tablespoons sugar

1 large egg

½ cup plus 2 tablespoons whole grain whole wheat flour

½ cup whey isolate protein powder

1 teaspoon baking powder

1 teaspoon baking soda

¼ teaspoon salt

¾ cup old-fashioned rolled oats

⅓ cup unsweetened applesauce (about the size of a single-serve portion)

¼ cup regular or mini semisweet chocolate chips

Preheat the oven to 350°F. Spray the muffin pan with cooking oil spray.

In a large bowl, mash the bananas well with a fork. Add the Splenda and sugar and mix well. Add the egg and mix well.

In a separate bowl, mix the flour, protein powder, baking powder, baking soda, salt, and oats. Add the dry ingredients to the wet and mix well. Add the applesauce and mix well. Add the chocolate chips and mix well.

Measure out 3 tablespoons of batter into 16 mini muffin cups for small muffins, or 6 tablespoons (100g) into 8 larger muffin cups. Bake for 20 to 25 minutes, depending on muffin size, or until a toothpick inserted in the center of a muffin comes out clean. Let cool for a few minutes in the pan, then pop out and store in a tightly closed container.

Per muffin: 104 calories, 5g protein (for mini muffins);
208 calories, 10g protein (for regular-size muffins)

Chocolate–Peanut Butter Protein Bars

Servings: 16 | Time to Table: 25 minutes (not including cooling) | Freezable

1 large egg

¼ cup sugar

½ cup Splenda

⅓ cup natural peanut butter

⅔ cup unsweetened applesauce
(about 2 single-serve portions)

¼ cup soy flour

½ cup whey isolate protein powder

⅓ cup unsweetened cocoa powder

½ cup old-fashioned rolled oats

½ cup quinoa

⅓ cup unsweetened shredded
coconut

Preheat the oven to 375°F. Line a 9 by 13-inch baking pan with parchment paper.

Toast raw quinoa in a dry pan over medium heat for about 5 minutes, until popping and brown; set aside.

Combine the egg, sugar, Splenda, peanut butter, and applesauce in a large bowl. In another bowl, combine the flour, protein powder, and unsweetened cocoa. Add to the wet ingredients and stir until well combined. Add the oats, quinoa, and coconut. Mix until well combined. Spread mixture evenly in the pan.

Bake for 15 minutes, until set.

Allow to cool completely in the pan before inverting onto a cutting board and peeling off the parchment paper. Cut into 16 bars. Wrap individual bars in plastic wrap and freeze in an airtight container or a heavy-duty resealable plastic bag.

Per bar: 140 calories, 7g protein

For school-safe bars, substitute soy-nut butter for peanut butter or remove altogether and reduce the baking time by 3 minutes.

Amazing Apple-Granola Bars

Servings: 16 | Time to Table: 40 minutes (not including cooling) | Freezable

¼ cup packed light brown sugar

2 tablespoons Splenda

¼ cup wheat germ

½ cup whey isolate protein powder (we use vanilla flavor, but any flavor will do)

½ cup quinoa flour

¼ cup flax seeds

¼ cup roasted shelled sunflower seeds

¼ cup roasted shelled pumpkin seeds

1½ cups old-fashioned rolled oats

1 large egg

¼ cup honey

1 teaspoon ground cinnamon

⅓ cup unsweetened applesauce (about the size of a single-serve portion)

1 large apple (I like Granny Smith or McIntosh), peeled, cored, and chopped

¾ cup coarsely chopped dried apples

¾ cup crisped rice cereal

Preheat the oven to 400°F. Line a 9 by 13-inch baking pan with parchment paper.

In a large bowl, combine the brown sugar, Splenda, wheat germ, protein powder, quinoa flour, flax seeds, sunflower seeds, pumpkin seeds, and rolled oats.

In a separate bowl, combine the egg, honey, cinnamon, and applesauce. Add to the dry mixture and stir until evenly moist. Add the chopped fresh and dried apples and the crisped rice and mix gently. Spread the mixture evenly in the baking pan.

Bake for 30 minutes or until firm and lightly browned on top.

Remove from the oven and invert onto a cutting board. Peel off the parchment paper. Allow to cool for 30 minutes before cutting into 16 bars.

When fully cooled, wrap individual bars in plastic wrap and freeze in an airtight container or a heavy-duty resealable plastic bag.

Per bar: 176 calories, 11g protein

Homemade Nut-Free Granola

Eat this by itself as a snack or use 2 tablespoons (65 calories, 3g protein) in the Yogurt Parfait that follows. I make this in a convection oven with an internal fan. If you have only a regular oven (no fan), it will take a little longer to get dry and crisp.

Servings: 10 (¼ cup each) | Time to Table: 35 minutes (not including cooling)

Canola oil cooking spray, optional

2 tablespoons water

1 tablespoon brown sugar

1 tablespoon honey

⅓ cup whey isolate protein
   powder (I use vanilla flavor,
   presweetened with Splenda)

1 cup old-fashioned rolled oats

1 cup textured vegetable protein

⅓ cup unsweetened applesauce

Preheat a convection oven to 350°F. Line a baking sheet with aluminum foil and spray the foil with cooking spray. Or use nonstick aluminum foil.

In a small cup, combine the water, brown sugar, and honey. Mix until dissolved.

In a medium bowl, combine the protein powder, oats, and textured vegetable protein. Add the applesauce and the honey–brown sugar mix. Stir until evenly moistened.

Spread the mixture on the baking sheet and bake for 10 minutes. Remove from the oven and use a spatula to turn the mixture over. Bake for another 5 to 10 minutes before removing from the oven and breaking it up with your hands (be careful, as it will be very hot). Return to the oven and bake for another 10 minutes or until crisp. Watch closely during the last 5 minutes of baking, as it can burn.

Remove from the oven and let cool. When completely cool, store in an airtight container. You may wish to break it up into smaller bits before storing.

Per ¼ cup: 101 calories, 9g protein

Yogurt Parfait

Servings: 1 | Time to Table: 3 minutes

½ cup plain fat-free Greek-style
    yogurt
1 teaspoon Splenda
1 teaspoon vanilla extract

⅓ cup chopped strawberries
3 tablespoons Homemade
    Nut-Free Granola

Combine the yogurt with the Splenda and vanilla. Stir in the strawberries and granola. Enjoy!

Per serving: 185 calories, 20g protein

Nut-Free Protein Granola Bars

Servings: 16 | Time to Table: 1 hour | Freezable

¼ cup brown sugar

¼ cup Splenda

¼ cup wheat germ

¼ cup flax seeds

1 teaspoon ground cinnamon

½ cup whole wheat flour

½ cup whey isolate protein powder (we use vanilla, but any flavor will do)

½ teaspoon kosher salt

2 cups old-fashioned rolled oats

¼ cup shelled sunflower seeds

¼ cup roasted shelled pumpkin seeds

¼ cup dried cranberries

1 large egg

⅓ cup mashed banana (roughly 1 medium banana)

1 teaspoon vanilla extract

¼ cup canola oil

¼ cup honey

¼ cup unsweetened applesauce

¾ cup crisped rice cereal

Preheat the oven to 400°F. Line a baking pan with parchment paper.

In a large bowl, combine the brown sugar, Splenda, wheat germ, flax seeds, cinnamon, whole wheat flour, protein powder, and salt. Add oats, sunflower seeds, pumpkin seeds, and dried cranberries.

In a separate bowl, combine the egg, mashed banana, vanilla, canola oil, honey, and applesauce. Add to the dry ingredients and mix well, until evenly moistened. Add the crisped rice and mix gently.

Spread the mixture evenly in the baking pan. Bake for 30 minutes or until firm and lightly browned on top.

Remove from the oven and invert onto a cutting board. Peel off the parchment paper. Allow to cool for 30 minutes before cutting into 16 bars.

When fully cooled, wrap individual bars in plastic wrap and freeze in an airtight container or a heavy-duty resealable plastic bag.

Per bar: 188 calories, 11g protein

Virtually Zero Effort Cottage Cheese and Fruit to the Rescue

Servings: 1 | Time to Table: 10 seconds to 1 minute

1 peach, pitted and chopped, or ½   ½ cup 1% fat cottage cheese
cup sliced peaches in juice

Add the peach to the cottage cheese. Enjoy.

Per serving: 133 calories, 15g protein (with fresh peaches);
144 calories, 15g protein (with sliced peaches in juice)

Know Your Nuts!

Here's the thing about nuts: they are not all created equal! The way they are processed—blanched, roasted, dry roasted, toasted, salted, unsalted, seasoned—can make a huge difference to calories, but even from the get-go, some nuts are higher in protein. So no matter what your nut of choice is, just make sure you know what they're worth.

Here is the breakdown, from "best" to "worst" from a caloric and protein snacking perspective using dry roasted nuts.

Nut (dry roasted)	Calories per 1-oz portion*	Protein per 1-oz portion
Soy nuts	135	11.9
Pumpkin seeds (shelled)	157	9.9
Peanuts	176	7.1
Walnuts	185	7.2
Almonds	179	6.6
Pistachios	171	6.4
Sunflower seeds (shelled)	175	5.8
Cashews	172	4.6
Hazelnuts/Filberts	183	4.3
Brazil nuts	201	4.2
Pecans	213	2.9

*Recently, the calorie content of nuts has been called into question, and it's possible that most nuts contain fewer calories than those provided in this list.

LUNCHES AND DINNERS

Stacey's Hide-the-Vegetables Pasta Sauce

Servings: 14 (1 cup each) | Time to Table: 1 hour to 1 hour 15 minutes (mostly unattended)

1 medium head cauliflower, trimmed and cut into florets

3 large Swiss chard leaves, stems discarded

2 stalks celery

15 to 20 white mushrooms, chopped

2 medium zucchini, stems trimmed

1 large red onion, peeled

4 cloves garlic, peeled and minced

Canola oil cooking spray

Two 28-ounce cans no-salt-added crushed tomatoes

1 teaspoon sugar

1 teaspoon freshly ground black pepper

2 teaspoons dried basil

2 teaspoons dried oregano

½ to 1 teaspoon salt, to taste

Bring an inch or two of water to a boil in a deep, large pot. Place a steamer rack in the pot, add the cauliflower, cover, and steam until quite tender (10 to 15 minutes, depending on the size of the florets).

While the cauliflower is cooking, coarsely chop the Swiss chard, celery, white mushrooms, zucchini, and onion. Mince the garlic.

Remove the cauliflower and set aside to drain, still in the steamer basket. Pour out any remaining water, and wipe the pot dry with paper towels. Spray the bottom of the pot with cooking spray and place over medium heat. Add the onion and garlic and cook, stirring occasionally, until transparent, about 5 minutes. Add the celery, Swiss chard, zucchini, and mushrooms. Cover and cook for 15 to 20 minutes, until softened (everything will cook faster with the cover on), stirring every few minutes.

(continued on next page)

Once the vegetables are well cooked, remove from the heat, drain in a colander, and return to the pot. Add the cauliflower, tomatoes, sugar, black pepper, basil, and oregano. Stir well and simmer over low heat for 30 minutes.

Puree in the pot using a handheld immersion blender. Or let cool until lukewarm and, working in batches, puree in a food processor or blender. Season to taste with salt. Pour the sauce into ½-, 1-, and 2-cup plastic containers and cover. Store in the fridge for up to 3 days, or freeze for longer storage.

Per cup (14 cups total per recipe): 93 calories, 5g protein

Gord's Lasagna

Named after Yoni's patient Gord who, when he smelled this lasagna re-heating in Yoni's office, knocked on Yoni's door to request the recipe. Serve with salad and light dressing. Freeze in individual portions for easy microwave reheating.

Servings: 12 | Time to Table: 1 hour 15 minutes (mostly unattended) | Freezable

1 cup textured vegetable protein (TVP; available at bulk food stores)

16 whole grain whole wheat lasagna noodles

5 cups Stacey's Hide-the-Vegetables Pasta Sauce (page 293)

1 pound low-fat mozzarella cheese, shredded

In a small pot, bring 1 cup water to a boil. Add the TVP, stir to mix, cover, and let it sit for at least 10 minutes to rehydrate.

Meanwhile, preheat the oven to 400°F and bring a large pot of water to a boil.

Add the lasagna noodles to the boiling water and cook according to the package directions for the minimum stated time. Drain in a colander and rinse with warm water to stop the cooking.

Combine the TVP with the pasta sauce. Spread about 1 cup of sauce on the bottom of a 9 by 13-inch baking pan. Place 4 noodles in a single layer and top with another cup of sauce and ¼ of the cheese. Repeat for all four layerings: noodles, sauce, and cheese, ending with a layer of cheese on top.

Bake 40 minutes, or until golden brown on top and heated through. Allow to cool for 5 to 10 minutes, then cut into 12 portions.

Per serving: 284 calories, 21g protein

Easy Eggplant Parmesan

Serve with a lightly dressed side salad. Freeze in individual portions for easy microwave reheating.

Servings: 8 | Time to Table: 45 to 55 minutes | Freezable

2 large eggplants

1 pound part-skim mozzarella cheese, shredded

5 cups Stacey's Hide-the-Vegetables Pasta Sauce (page 293)

Cut off and discard the stems of the eggplants. Slice each eggplant from top to bottom (lengthwise) into slices about ½-inch thick. Place the eggplants back together by stacking the pieces, and put on a paper towel–lined microwaveable plate. Cover each eggplant with a dry paper towel.

Microwave on high power for approximately 15 minutes, or until soft to the touch. Let cool for several minutes before handling. Discard the paper towels.

While the eggplants are in the microwave, preheat the oven to 400°F.

Spread 1 cup of sauce across the bottom of a 9 by 13-inch baking pan. Place slices of eggplant in a single layer atop the sauce, covering the bottom of the pan, as you would with noodles for lasagna. Cover with more sauce, then 1 cup of the cheese. Repeat until all the eggplant and sauce are used up, ending with cheese covering the top.

Bake for 30 to 40 minutes, until the top begins to brown. Allow a few minutes to cool before dividing into 8 portions.

Per serving: 263 calories, 21g protein (not including salad)

Savory Four-Cheese Crêpe "Manicotti"

Servings: 7 | Time to Table: 1 hour | Freezable

For the filling

Canola oil cooking spray

¼ onion, chopped

2 teaspoons minced garlic

One 15-ounce container part-skim ricotta cheese

1½ cups grated part-skim mozzarella cheese

⅓ cup grated Parmesan cheese

4 ounces light cream cheese

½ teaspoon dried oregano

½ teaspoon dried basil

½ teaspoon ground black pepper

One 10-ounce package frozen chopped spinach, cooked and drained, or 1 pound fresh spinach, cooked, drained, and chopped

For the crêpes

1 large egg

1 teaspoon baking powder

½ teaspoon dried oregano

½ teaspoon dried basil

1 teaspoon olive oil

¾ cup whole grain whole wheat flour

1½ cups water

Canola oil cooking spray

2½ cups Stacey's Hide-the-Vegetables Pasta Sauce (page 293)

To make the filling: Lightly spray a nonstick pan with cooking spray and place over medium heat. Add the onion and garlic and cook, stirring occasionally, until soft and translucent. Remove from the heat.

In a large bowl, combine the ricotta, mozzarella, Parmesan, cream cheese, oregano, basil, and pepper. Add the cooked onions and garlic and the spinach, and stir to mix thoroughly.

Preheat the oven to 400°F.

To make the crêpes: In a separate bowl, whisk together all the ingredients until well blended. The consistency should be like that of thin

(continued on next page)

cream. Heat a medium nonstick frying pan over medium heat and spray it lightly with cooking spray. When the pan is hot, ladle in approximately ¼ cup of batter, tilting the pan to evenly coat the bottom.

When the edges begin to curl off the pan, use your fingers to pull the crêpe up from the pan and flip it over. Cook for another 30 to 40 seconds on the other side before removing the crêpe. Repeat until all the batter is used up, making 7 crêpes.

Spread ½ cup (130g) of the filling down the middle of each crêpe, then roll up the crêpe so that it is sealed and will not open while cooking.

Spread 1 cup of pasta sauce on the bottom of a 2-quart oblong baking pan. Place the crêpes side by side in the pan, seam side down, on top of the sauce. Top with the remaining 1½ cups sauce. Bake for 30 to 40 minutes, until slightly browned and the filling and sauce are bubbling.

Per filled crêpe: 305 calories, 21g protein

Did Someone Say Pizza?

This recipe makes enough dough for six 10- to 12-inch pizzas (depending on how thick or thin you roll them), 6 slices each. The dough will keep in the fridge (covered with plastic wrap) for up to 2 weeks, or in the freezer (double-wrapped in plastic) for longer. The sauce makes approximately 2 cups, and we use ⅓ cup per pizza. If you have the freezer space, you can make all 6 pizzas, freeze them unbaked, then bake as you want them. No need for store-bought frozen or take-out pizza ever again!

Servings: 36 slices (6 pizzas, 6 slices each) | Time to Table Once Prepared: 15 to 20 minutes

For the no-knead dough

2¾ cups warm water

1 tablespoon sugar

¾ teaspoon kosher salt

¼ cup olive oil

1½ tablespoons quick-rise bread machine yeast

6 cups whole grain whole wheat flour

½ cup unflavored whey isolate protein powder

For the sauce

One 28-ounce can no-salt-added crushed tomatoes

1 tablespoon sugar

1 teaspoon dried oregano

1 teaspoon dried basil

¾ teaspoon garlic powder

¾ teaspoon freshly ground black pepper

½ teaspoon dried onion flakes

Additional toppings of your choice, optional (don't forget to calculate their additional calories)

2¼ pounds part-skim mozzarella, shredded

To make the dough: Pour the warm water into a large bowl. Add the sugar, salt, olive oil, and yeast. Mix with a spoon until the yeast is

(continued on next page)

dissolved. Add the flour and protein powder, and then mix with a spoon or your hands to fully incorporate the flour. Cover with a clean kitchen towel and let it rest and rise at room temperature for 2 hours.

To make the sauce: While the dough is rising, in a saucepan, combine all the ingredients. Bring to a boil, then simmer on low heat for 10 to 15 minutes for the flavors to blend.

To make the pizzas: Preheat the oven to 525°F and line a baking sheet with parchment paper.

Divide the dough into 6 equal pieces. For each pizza, roll or pat 1 piece of dough on the baking sheet into a 10- to 12-inch diameter circle. (Store the remaining dough in the fridge or freezer.) Spread with ⅓ cup of the sauce. If desired, scatter with additional topping. Sprinkle with ⅙ of the shredded cheese (about 6 ounces). Bake for 5 to 10 minutes, ideally on a pizza stone that has been preheating in the oven, or until the edge of the crust is browned and the cheese is melted and bubbling. Let cool briefly, then cut into 6 slices and enjoy!

Per slice (with cheese and sauce only): 192 calories, 13g protein

Way Simple Whole Wheat Tortilla Wraps

These wraps serve as the base of a number of recipes to follow and make buying wraps a wholly unnecessary exercise.

Servings: 10 | Time to Table: 30 minutes

2 cups whole grain whole wheat flour

¼ cup unseasoned instant mashed potato flakes

1 teaspoon baking powder

½ teaspoon salt

2 tablespoons olive oil

¾ cup warm water

Whole grain whole wheat flour for rolling

In a medium bowl, stir together the flour, potato flakes, baking powder, and salt. Add the olive oil and mix well. Add the water and mix with your hands until all the dry ingredients have been incorporated and the dough holds together in a ball. Leave to rest, covered with a clean kitchen towel, for 15 to 20 minutes.

Heat a large heavy frying pan (cast-iron is best) on medium heat for 5 minutes.

Divide the dough into 10 equal balls. Roll out each ball as thin as possible. I roll them between a floured silicone baking mat and parchment paper, but you can also use 2 pieces of parchment paper.

Transfer a dough round to the heated pan and cook until bubbles form, 30 to 60 seconds. Flip to the second side for another 30 to 60 seconds. Remove from the pan. Continue until all the dough is cooked, stacking the wraps on a plate. Store any leftovers in a heavy-duty resealable plastic bag in the freezer (not in the fridge). These reheat nicely in the oven or in a pan on low temperature.

Per wrap: 126 calories, 4g protein

Guaca-Moly!

Servings: 18 | Time to Table: 30 minutes (but preps in 2)

2 ripe avocados, split and pitted

1 small tomato, finely chopped

1 large chipotle chile in adobo, minced (more for more heat and smoke)

½ cup finely chopped red onion

1½ tablespoons fresh lemon juice

¼ teaspoon garlic powder

Scoop the avocado flesh into a medium bowl and mash with a fork. Add all the remaining ingredients and stir together. Cover with plastic wrap and let sit in the fridge for 30 minutes before devouring! And don't forget to add the pits to the mix to keep the guacamole from turning brown.

Per 1½ tablespoons: 18 calories, no protein to speak of

Cornflake Encrusted Whitefish

You can serve these to kids in place of boxed fish sticks. They also are great in the Fabulous Fish Tacos that follow!

Servings: 12 | Time to Table: 30 minutes

Canola oil cooking spray
1 pound whitefish fillets
(usually 3 fillets hake, haddock,
tilapia, or sole)

⅓ cup whole wheat flour
¼ cup pasteurized egg whites,
or 1 large egg, lightly beaten
2 cups cornflakes

Preheat the oven to 400°F. Line a baking sheet with parchment paper and spray the paper lightly with cooking spray. Cut each fillet into quarters.

Spread the flour on one plate, place the egg whites in a medium bowl, and hand-crush the cornflakes and spread on another plate. Using a fork, pick up a piece of fish and coat it completely in flour, then in egg white, then press into the cornflakes on all sides.

Place the fish pieces on the baking sheet. Repeat with the remaining fish. Lightly spray the top of all the fish with cooking spray.

Bake for 15 to 20 minutes, flipping once. The fillets will be crisp and golden brown when finished.

Per quarter fillet: 76 calories, 9g protein

Fabulous Fish Tacos

These are great as they are, or you can add hot sauce or salsa to spice things up. You might also consider squeezing on some fresh lemon juice.

Servings: 1 | Time to Table: Will vary depending on how much of various ingredients need cooking

1 Way Simple Whole Wheat Tortilla Wrap (page 301), cooked

2 pieces Cornflake Encrusted Whitefish (preceding recipe)

1½ tablespoons Guaca-Moly! (page 302)

1 tablespoon shredded low-fat cheddar cheese

2 tablespoons refried beans, warm

1½ tablespoons light sour cream

Top the wrap with the fish, then top the fish with everything else. Eat while it's all hot!

Per fish taco: 352 calories, 26g protein

Goat Cheese, Cranberry, Walnut, and Beet Salad

Servings: 1 | Time to Table: 5 minutes

2½ cups torn red leaf lettuce

9 or 10 cherry tomatoes, halved or
left whole

½ small red bell pepper, diced

1 ounce soft goat cheese, crumbled

¼ cup walnuts, coarscly chopped

2 tablespoons dried cranberries

1 small roasted or canned beet,
diced

Combine all the ingredients and top with the dressing of your choice.

Per serving: 395 calories, 19g protein (without dressing)
By reducing the walnuts from ¼ cup to 2 tablespoons, you can
reduce the per serving amounts to 327 calories, 15g protein

Tuna Sandwiches "with a Twist"

Servings: 2 | Time to Table: 10 minutes

½ ripe avocado

One 5-ounce can light tuna in
  water, drained

1 teaspoon lemon juice

1 pinch salt

1 pinch freshly ground black
  pepper

4 slices whole grain whole wheat
  bread, toasted if desired

2 lettuce leaves

4 slices tomato

Alfalfa sprouts or other raw
  vegetables, optional

Mash the avocado in a small bowl. Add the tuna, lemon juice, salt, and
pepper and mix. Divide the tuna mixture between slices of bread. Top
each with 1 lettuce leaf, 2 tomato slices, and sprouts or other desired veg-
gie toppings (and, of course, the second slice of bread). Cut into halves or
quarters, and enjoy!

Per sandwich: 298 calories, 23g protein

Truly Fantastic Fish Soup

Instead of the water and fish bouillon, you can use fresh fish stock—something you might be able to buy from your fishmonger. I serve this with a slice of fresh baked whole wheat baguette—yum! If you have any leftovers, freeze in 2-cup microwaveable containers to enjoy again later. Reheat gently so the fish doesn't get too overcooked.

Servings: 8 | Time to Table: 1 hour | Freezable

3 tablespoons olive oil

1 bulb fennel, stalks and leaves removed, thinly sliced

1 small red onion, peeled and chopped

3 large shallots, peeled and chopped

4 cloves garlic, peeled and minced

¾ teaspoon hot red pepper flakes

¼ cup tomato paste

One 28-ounce can diced tomatoes, with juice

1½ cups dry white wine

5 cups water

1 tablespoon fish bouillon powder or 2 fish bouillon cubes

1 bay leaf

1 pound skinless salmon fillet, cut into 1-inch cubes

1 pound skinless tilapia fillets, cut into 1-inch cubes

1 pound skinless rainbow trout fillets, cut into 1-inch cubes

Heat the olive oil in a large pot over medium heat. Add the fennel, onion, and shallots and cook, stirring occasionally, until the onion is translucent, 5 to 10 minutes.

Add the garlic and pepper flakes and cook for another 2 minutes.

Stir in the tomato paste, and then add the tomatoes with their juices, the wine, water, fish bouillon, and bay leaf. Cover and simmer for 30 minutes.

Add the fish and cook for another 5 minutes. Remove the bay leaf before serving.

Per 2-cup bowl: 310 calories, 38g protein

Perfectly Roasted Chicken

Enjoy with a fresh garden salad or other side dish! Leftovers? See the Crazy Good Chicken Taco Soup (page 310) and So-Simple Roast Chicken Sandwich (page 312) recipes that follow.

Servings: 8 | Time to Table: 1½ hours | Freezable (wrapped in several layers of plastic wrap)

One 4-pound whole chicken

Juice of ½ lemon (about 2 tablespoons)

½ teaspoon salt

2 teaspoons freshly ground black pepper

2 teaspoons paprika

1 teaspoon chicken bouillon powder

¼ cup water

Move the bottom oven rack as low as it will go (depending on the size of your oven, you may need to remove the upper racks). Preheat the oven to 350°F.

Remove and discard the innards from the chicken. Pat skin dry with paper towels.

Squeeze the lemon juice over the entire chicken, including the inside. Combine the salt, pepper, and paprika and sprinkle over the entire chicken, including the inside. Rub in as needed to form an even coat.

Combine the chicken bouillon and water to make a basting liquid.

Place the chicken on a vertical roasting stand (or an empty beer can), so that the chicken is standing upright (you can buy a vertical roaster in any BBQ store and many large department stores). Place the stand in a shallow roasting pan.

Place the chicken in the oven and roast for 1 hour and 15 minutes, basting every 20 minutes.

To ensure that the chicken is cooked through, use the "leg test," piercing the joint with a fork to see if the juices run clear, and twisting the leg to see if it moves easily. Or if you're unfamiliar with cooking a whole chicken, use an instant-read meat thermometer, which should read 180°F when stuck into the thigh (just don't stick it into bone). Transfer the chicken to a cutting board to rest for about 5 minutes. Discard the drippings. Carve the chicken into 8 pieces (2 legs, 2 thighs, 2 wings with some of the breast attached, and 2 breast halves).

Per average serving: 337 calories, 29g protein

Crazy Good Chicken Taco Soup

You can make this by cooking fresh chicken first. But it's great—and easy—with leftover roasted chicken!

Servings: 6 | Time to Table: 1 hour | Freezable

6 cups chicken stock or broth (preferably unsalted or low-sodium)

1 pound boneless, skinless chicken breast fillets or leftover cooked chicken breast, skin and bones removed

2 tablespoons canola oil

1 medium yellow onion, peeled and thinly sliced

2 cloves garlic, peeled and chopped

1 jalapeño pepper, chopped

One 28-ounce can whole peeled tomatoes

1 medium yellow onion, peeled and chopped

3 cloves garlic, peeled and minced

Freshly ground black pepper

⅔ cup fresh, frozen, or canned corn kernels (no salt added if using canned)

1 cup drained cooked black beans

1 cup water

1 tablespoon chopped fresh cilantro

Salt

Hand-crushed corn chips, for serving, optional

If using fresh chicken, in a large pot, bring the chicken stock to a boil. Add the raw chicken fillets, cover, reduce the heat, and simmer until the chicken is cooked through, about 10 minutes. Remove the chicken from the pot and allow to cool for a few minutes before shredding with your fingers or 2 forks. If using cooked chicken, just shred it.

For the "salsa," heat 1 tablespoon of the canola oil in a medium pan and add the sliced onion, chopped garlic, and jalapeño. Cook over medium heat, stirring occasionally, until soft, 5 to 10 minutes. Add the tomatoes with their juices and simmer for 10 to 15 minutes.

Transfer to a blender and puree until smooth. (Be careful blending hot food; fill the blender only partway, and hold the top down with a folded kitchen towel. Work in batches if necessary.) Set aside.

In the same pan, heat another tablespoon of oil over medium heat.

Add the chopped onion, minced garlic, and ½ teaspoon of the pepper. Cook until soft, 5 to 10 minutes.

Add the cooked onion mixture, "salsa," shredded chicken, corn, black beans, water, and cilantro to the chicken stock. Bring to a boil and simmer on low heat for 15 minutes. Add salt and pepper to taste. If you like, add a small amount (2 tablespoons/10g) of hand-crushed corn chips when serving. We don't tend to add salt if we're using corn chips.

Per 2-cup bowl (without chips): 249 calories, 26g protein

Per 2-cup bowl (with 2 tablespoons/10g chips): 301 calories, 26g protein

So-Simple Roast Chicken Sandwich

What could be simpler?

Servings: 1 | Time to Table: 2 minutes (max!)

1 tablespoon mayonnaise

2 slices whole grain whole wheat
    bread, plain or toasted

2½ ounces roasted chicken breast
    meat, pulled into small pieces

2 slices tomato

1 lettuce leaf

Spread the mayo on the bread, then build the sandwich with the remaining ingredients.

Per sandwich: 439 calories, 30g protein

If you use light mayonnaise, you'll save on the order of 50 calories.

Spicy Slow Cooker Chili

Be very careful if using habaneros—you might even want to wear disposable gloves when cutting them, and know that frying them can cause coughing fits and watery eyes. If you use the max of all the chiles, this will be super spicy!

Servings: 8 | Time to Table: At least 4 hours and up to 6 hours, mostly unattended
(plus 15 minutes preparation)

Canola oil cooking spray

1½ pounds ground turkey

1 large green bell pepper, chopped

1 large yellow onion, peeled and chopped

3 or 4 cloves garlic, peeled and minced

1 to 3 fresh habanero chiles, seeded and chopped, optional

One 28-ounce can no-salt-added diced tomatoes

18 ounces drained cooked black beans (rinsed if canned)

1 tablespoon brown sugar (loosely filled, not packed)

1 tablespoon chili powder

¼ cup dark beer, optional

3 dashes liquid smoke

2 to 4 chipotle chiles in adobo, coarsely chopped

One 4.4-ounce can New Mexico green chiles, drained, optional

Lightly spray a large pan with cooking spray and brown the turkey, using a spoon to break up big clumps. Drain the fat and juices and transfer the turkey to the slow cooker. Add all the remaining ingredients to the slow cooker and mix well. Cover and cook on high for 2 to 3 hours, then uncover and cook on low for another 2 to 3 hours, stirring occasionally, to reduce the liquid.

Per cup: 346 calories, 31g protein

Magnificent Mediterranean "Sausage" Wraps

Servings: 5 | Time to Table: 25 minutes (not including wraps dough)

1 teaspoon freshly ground black pepper

1 teaspoon ground cinnamon

1 teaspoon ground ginger

1 teaspoon ground cumin

1 teaspoon ground coriander

¼ teaspoon kosher salt

¼ teaspoon smoked paprika

1 pound lean ground turkey

½ recipe Way Simple Whole Wheat Tortilla Wraps (page 301), uncooked

Condiments of your choice (I like yellow mustard; Yoni likes mayonnaise and homemade spicy mango mustard)

Preheat the oven to 450°F. Place two heavy frying pans (not nonstick; cast-iron is best) on medium heat to preheat for 5 minutes.

In a medium bowl, mix together the pepper, cinnamon, ginger, cumin, coriander, salt, and paprika. Add the ground turkey meat and work in the spices evenly with your hands. Divide into five balls and roll by hand into sausages about 2 inches in diameter.

Place the sausages in one of the pans and cook on all sides until browned all over (about 40 seconds each side). Transfer the sausages to a baking sheet and bake for 8 minutes.

While the sausages are baking, divide the dough into five equal balls. Roll out each ball as thin as possible, to 5 to 6 inches in diameter. (I roll them between a silicone baking mat and parchment paper, but you can also use two pieces of parchment paper.)

Transfer a dough round to the other heated pan and cook until bubbles form, 30 to 60 seconds. Flip to the second side for another 30 to 60 seconds. Repeat with the remaining dough until all five wraps are cooked.

Place one sausage in each wrap and top with condiments. Roll and enjoy!

Per wrap (not including condiments): 267 calories, 20g protein

---

Invite-Guests-Over Mediterranean
Grilled Chicken and Vegetable Kebabs

If you want, you can marinate the chicken overnight, then add the vegetables the next day, about an hour before cooking. I usually make a double batch of the marinade and cut up an extra pound of the chicken breast to freeze together in a heavy-duty resealable plastic bag for later use. We use metal skewers, but wood or bamboo can be used as well; just make sure you soak them in water first for about 30 minutes. Safety note: *do not* baste the kebabs with leftover marinade, and do not use it as a sauce; food-borne illness is a terrible way to lose weight!

Servings: 6 | Time to Table: 30 minutes (not including marinating time)

For the marinade

¼ cup chopped scallions (green onions; use more of the whites than the greens)

¼ cup fresh chopped fresh parsley

¼ cup fresh chopped fresh cilantro

6 cloves garlic, peeled and minced

2 teaspoons smoked paprika

2 teaspoons ground cumin

¼ teaspoon cayenne pepper

½ teaspoon salt

½ cup olive oil

For the kebabs

1¼ pounds boneless, skinless chicken breast

1 large red bell pepper

1 large green bell pepper

2 medium zucchini

10 large white mushroom caps

1 medium red onion

For serving

1 cup quinoa

2 cups water

To make the marinade: Combine all the ingredients in a blender or food processor and puree until smooth.

(continued on next page)

To make the kebabs: Cut up the chicken breasts into chunks that won't fall off the skewers. Cut the red and green peppers in half and re-move the stems and seeds. Cut the peppers into medium-large chunks. Remove the ends from the zucchini and cut crosswise into 1- to 1½-inch slices. Wipe the mushroom caps clean with a damp paper towel, if neces-sary. Peel and quarter the onion.

Place the chicken and vegetables in a large heavy-duty resealable plas-tic bag or a large glass bowl. Add marinade and mix well, until all the vegetables and the chicken are well covered with marinade. Let sit in the fridge for 1 to 2 hours.

When you're almost ready to serve, heat the grill to high. Combine the quinoa and water in a saucepan, bring to a boil, cover, and simmer for about 15 minutes, until the water has been absorbed and the little quinoa tails unfurl. Keep warm.

Remove the vegetables and chicken from the marinade. Place pieces of vegetables and chicken on skewers and grill over high heat until the chicken is cooked through, about 15 minutes, turning occasionally.

Serve over quinoa and enjoy!

Per serving: 402 calories, 27g protein

Vegan Tofu, Sweet Potato, and Chickpea Curry

Freeze in individual portions for easy microwave reheating.

Servings: 8 | Time to Table: 35 minutes | Freezable

Canola oil cooking spray
1 medium red onion, peeled and
   chopped
2 cloves garlic, peeled and minced
2 teaspoons Thai red curry paste
1 large sweet potato (about
   1 pound), peeled and cubed
One 14-ounce can chickpeas,
   drained and rinsed
One 14-ounce can coconut milk
½ cup low-sodium vegetable broth
2 tablespoons low-sodium soy
   sauce
1 packed tablespoon brown sugar
1 tablespoon curry powder
1 large red bell pepper, thinly
   sliced
1 pound firm tofu, cubed
¼ cup chopped fresh cilantro
2 tablespoons lime juice
2 cups cooked brown rice, for
   serving

Lightly spray a large nonstick frying pan with cooking spray and place over medium heat. Add the onion, garlic, and Thai curry paste and cook, stirring occasionally, until the onion is soft.

Add the sweet potato, chickpeas, coconut milk, vegetable broth, soy sauce, brown sugar, and curry powder. Bring to a boil, then reduce the heat to low, partially cover, and simmer until the sweet potato is almost tender, about 12 minutes.

Add the red pepper and tofu to the pan and cook for another 2 to 5 minutes, until the tofu is heated through. Remove from heat. Stir in the fresh chopped cilantro and lime juice.

Serve over brown rice.

Per serving: 459 calories, 18g protein

Spectacular Sweet and Spicy Chicken and Broccoli Stir-Fry

For a vegan option, substitute 3 pounds firm tofu for the chicken. The calories will remain approximately the same, but the protein will be roughly halved.

Servings: 6 | Time to Table: 40 minutes (including cooking rice)

2 pounds boneless, skinless chicken breast

6 to 8 scallions (green onions), thinly sliced, whites only

6 Thai green chiles, chopped

¼ cup chopped fresh basil

2 teaspoons minced garlic, divided in two

2 teaspoons minced ginger, divided in two

¼ cup sugar

2 tablespoons low-sodium soy sauce

2 tablespoons dry sherry

4 tablespoons sesame oil, divided in two

2 teaspoons cornstarch

2 teaspoons hot red pepper flakes

2 large heads broccoli

2 tablespoons olive oil

2 tablespoons hoisin sauce

½ cup water

5 cups cooked brown rice, for serving

Cut the chicken into bite-size pieces and place in a large bowl. Add the scallions, chiles, basil, 1 teaspoon of the garlic, 1 teaspoon of the ginger, the sugar, soy sauce, sherry, 2 tablespoons of the sesame oil, the cornstarch, and red pepper flakes, mix well, and set aside.

Cut the broccoli florets into bite-size pieces. Remove the ends and peel the stems, and cut into ½-inch-thick pieces. Add the remaining 1 teaspoon garlic and 1 teaspoon ginger to the broccoli.

Heat the olive oil and the remaining 2 tablespoons sesame oil in a wok over high heat and add the chicken mixture. Stir-fry until the chicken is cooked through. Add the hoisin sauce and broccoli to the pan and sprinkle with the water, cover, and steam the broccoli until bright green. Remove the pan and set aside.

Toss to combine and serve immediately over brown rice.

Per serving: 483 calories, 38g protein

Vegetarian Chimichangas!

These can be eaten plain as is after baking, or you can also bake them with cheese on top, and/or top with salsa, guacamole, or sour cream. Freeze in individual portions for easy microwave reheating.

Servings: 17 | Time to Table: 25 minutes | Freezable

Canola oil cooking spray

1 cup chopped red onion

6 cloves garlic, peeled and minced

One 4.4-ounce can diced green chiles

1 medium ripe avocado, split, pitted, peeled, and diced

1½ cups low-sodium salsa

1½ cups grated low-fat cheddar cheese

One 16-ounce can low-sodium refried beans

6¼ cups cooked black beans

2 cups cooked brown rice

2 teaspoons ground cumin

2 teaspoons chili powder

3 tablespoons low-fat Greek-style yogurt

17 Way Simple Whole Wheat Tortilla Wraps (page 301), cooked

Preheat the oven to 400°F. Lightly spray a large baking sheet with cooking spray.

Lightly spray a nonstick frying pan with cooking spray. Add the onion and garlic and cook, stirring occasionally, until the onion is soft. Add the green chiles with their juices and cook for another 3 to 4 minutes before removing from the heat.

In a large bowl, combine the avocado, salsa, cheese, refried beans, black beans, brown rice, cumin, and chili powder with the contents from the pan. Mix gently but thoroughly.

Place ½ cup filling in the center of a each wrap and fold as if sealing a box. Place the packages seam side down on the baking sheet. Bake for 10 minutes.

Per ½-cup filling: 150 calories, 9g protein

Per filled wrap (not including toppings): 280 calories, 15g protein

RESOURCES

Books

What to Eat by Dr. Marion Nestle
An aisle-by-aisle guide to supermarket shopping by one of the world's foremost authorities in nutrition. Although this is not a diet book, Dr. Nestle seeks to help you understand how to shop in a complicated marketplace. She covers topics such as which organic fruits and vegetables you should consider buying, how to shop healthfully for fish, and what the different types of labels mean, and all in all makes you a far more savvy shopper.

The No-Sweat Exercise Plan by Dr. Harvey Simon
From Harvard, here's a healthy guide on how to increase the exercise in your life. Of course, you can also just keep in mind my eight-word exercise manifesto: "Some is good. More is better. Everything counts."

The Body Image Workbook by Dr. Thomas Cash
Dr. Cash, an expert on body image, wrote this book as a self-help guide for folks who suffer with body image distress. He reports that in clinical trials, individuals who complete his workbook significantly improve their body image satisfaction and decrease their body image distress. That's not to say you'll read this book and want to mow your lawn in a thong, but it may just make you comfortable enough in your own skin to be able to more richly enjoy your life. Be forewarned, it's an aptly titled book with a great many self-exploration exercises. Should you decide to buy and work through it, I'd recommend that you use a separate notepad to record your answers and your diarizing, as many of my patients who've used the book have gone back through it a second time down the road, and it'll work better if you don't have your old answers skewing your thoughts.

Mindless Eating by Dr. Brian Wansink

This is a fascinating book. Dr. Wansink's career has been built on studying the mindless eating cues that influence many of our 200 daily dietary decisions. From the size of bowls and packages, to how many people we eat with, to the impact of front-of-package statements such as "low-fat," Dr. Wansink's book reads like an exposé of brain-food interactions we didn't even know were there. More important, Dr. Wansink's work will help open your eyes to significant sources of mindless calories, as well as provide you with a battle plan to protect yourself.

Useful Web Resources

The Diet Fix (www.TheDietFix.com)

Tools and resources useful to you as readers of this book. Resting energy expenditure calculators, exercise expenditure calculators, a forum where you can ask me and other experts questions, as well as printable food diary pages and more.

Weighty Matters (www.weightymatters.ca)

My daily blog covering topics ranging from food advertising to nutrition and obesity policy to exercise and weight management. Here you'll also find links to some of my favorite bloggers.

CalorieKing (www.calorieking.com)

Provides a huge database of calories, but most important, many different measurement options in a drop-down format.

My Fitness Pal (www.myfitnesspal.com)

Our office's food diary app of choice. Also has smartphone and iPad apps that seamlessly integrate with one another. Keep your eyes peeled for The Diet Fix Diary app.

Fitocracy (www.fitocracy.com)

Think food diary, but for exercise, combined with Facebook and with built-in rewards/achievements, and you've got Fitocracy. Terrifically friendly and encouraging users are what really make this website shine. Smartphone apps to track when you're on the run just add to its ease of use.

Oh Don't Forget (ohdontforget.com)
An invaluable service that allows you to set up reminders to be sent via text message to your cell phone. Remind yourself to shop, snack, or exercise. The free online service allows for only one reminder to be set up at a time, but drop a few dollars and you can set it up to send as many reminders as you want, and even send them recurrently. (Of course, you could also simply use your phone's reminder app, yet, strangely, many find texts to be more compelling.)

Useful Computer Programs

MasterCook, Living Cookbook, and *MacGourmet*
The first two are PC recipe databases that allow you not only to store your recipes, but with simple clicks to also determine caloric and nutritional information. Of the two, MasterCook's interface is less refined, but its price is tough to beat. *Living Cookbook* offers a free downloadable 30-day trial at www.livingcook book.com.

   If you're a Mac user, then I'm told *MacGourmet* is the way to go (www.mac gourmet.com)

Useful Smartphone Apps

MyFitnessPal
Our office dietitian's food diary app of choice. My only complaint is that there's no means with which to track the times that you're eating.

Fooducate
Fooducate is a free app designed by Hemi Weingarten and his Fooducate team. It's available only for the U.S. market. Use it to scan bar codes in the supermarket to learn about nutritional content and to be given healthier alternatives.

Nike+
Nike+ is my running app of choice. It'll allow you to tap into your Facebook and Twitter friends for support while walking, running, or cycling, and it integrates with a wonderfully designed online site to track your progress. Celebrities and sports heroes will applaud your progress.

RunKeeper

More popular than Nike+, and it integrates directly with Fitocracy. Not a regular user myself, I can't comment much, though my friends who use it are big fans.

Zombies Run!

If you need an extra boost of motivation, this app will enhance your running with an interactive story line. A great way to have more fun on your runs!

ACKNOWLEDGMENTS

It's rare in life to be given an opportunity to publicly thank people for what they've done. While I can't pass that up, no doubt there are dozens, if not hundreds, of people who have had profound impacts on me over the years, and I consider myself truly fortunate to have met them all. This list I'll keep to the truly transformational. I want to thank my parents for their generosity and patience in providing me with the freedom to pursue any and all of my dreams; Bill Gregg and Judy Irvine at the University of Toronto, without whom I'd almost certainly not be a physician today; my patients, for teaching me more than I could have ever learned in medical school; my brother-in-law Lorne Segal for helping to keep the lights on; Holly Bodger for being the world's sagest bookwriting friend; Foundry Literary + Media's Yfat Reiss Gendell for taking a chance on an unknown; Leah Miller and the rest of the gang at Harmony Books for their counsel, enthusiasm, and trust; and lastly, of course, my unbelievable wife, Stacey, who—cliché or not—is the only reason any of this was possible.

INDEX

ABOUT THE AUTHOR

Dr. Yoni Freedhoff, MD, CCFP, graduated with honors from the University of Toronto Faculty of Medicine, where he received the Betty Stewart Sisam Award as the graduating student who "has shown the greatest human understanding and care for the welfare and health of patients." Widely considered to be Canada's most outspoken obesity expert, Dr. Freedhoff writes a weekly column in *U.S. News & World Report*'s online Eat + Run edition that is regularly the most shared on the site, and he writes periodically on issues of health, weight management, and fitness for a variety of publications, including *Psychology Today* and the *Huffington Post,* and daily on his award-winning blog *Weighty Matters.* He is also an assistant professor in the Faculty of Medicine at the University of Ottawa and a sought-after international speaker.